EXERCISES IN DIAGNOSTIC RADIOLOGY

CHEST, ABDOMEN, BONE
and
CLINICAL SKILLS
A Problem-Based Text

EXERCISES IN DIAGNOSTIC RADIOLOGY

CHEST, ABDOMEN, BONE and CLINICAL SKILLS
A Problem-Based Text

Judith Korek Amorosa, M.D.
Clinical Professor of Radiology
Director of Medical Education
Department of Radiology
Robert Wood Johnson Medical
    School
New Brunswick, New Jersey

Robert A. Novelline, M.D.
Director of Emergency Radiology
Massachusetts General Hospital
Associate Professor of Radiology
Harvard Medical School
Boston, Massachusetts

Lucy Frank Squire, M.D.
Professor of Radiology
State University of New York
Downstate Medical Center
Brooklyn, New York

W. B. SAUNDERS COMPANY

Harcourt Brace Jovanovich, Inc.

Philadelphia   London   Toronto   Montreal   Sydney   Tokyo

W. B. SAUNDERS COMPANY
Harcourt Brace Jovanovich, Inc.

The Curtis Center
Independence Square West
Philadelphia, Pennsylvania 19106

Library of Congress Cataloging-in-Publication Data

Amorosa, Judith K.

Exercises in diagnostic radiology: chest, abdomen, bone and clinical skills: a problem-based text / Judith K. Amorosa, Robert A. Novelline, Lucy Frank Squire.—3rd ed.

p.   cm.

Rev. ed. of: Exercises in diagnostic radiology / Lucy Frank Squire [et al.]. Combined 2nd ed. c1982.

ISBN 0–7216–3129–0

1. Diagnosis, Radioscopic—Programmed instruction.
   I. Novelline, Robert A.   II. Squire, Lucy Frank
   III. Title.

[DNLM: 1. Radiography—programmed instruction. WN 18 A524e]

RC78.A659   1992

616.07′57—dc20
DNLM/DLC   91–27915

EXERCISES IN DIAGNOSTIC RADIOLOGY:
CHEST, ABDOMEN, BONE AND CLINICAL SKILLS   ISBN 0–7216–3129–0

We dedicate this book to our parents
Lorant J. and Klara Korek
Joseph A. and Emma Anita Novelline
Leslie C. and Ethelwyn Frank

Preface for Students and Teachers

This book is intended to function in medical training and during the first year of graduate training as a self-testing, self-instructional supplement to *Fundamentals of Radiology* (LFS, RAN). The exercises on the chest, abdomen and bone are based on the assumption that the student will have read the corresponding sections of the textbook.

The reader would not be entertained by guessing the point of an exercise immediately; that should be evident only as he reviews it after it has been completed and the answers have been studied. Therefore, students are urged to follow directions closely and to work through the book from beginning to end. The exercises are progressive and often interlocked.

Readers should make a practice of tipping and folding the pages, as directed, so that the posteroanterior and lateral films are viewed together, as the layout arrangement provides. The reader is also urged to study with a tablet at hand upon which he writes down his answers before turning to the answer page that follows.

A book of exercises should be a close reproduction of the random nature of medical practice. Therefore, this book is composed of groups of two or three patients presenting with similar symptoms and having different disease conditions and roentgen findings. At the same time, we have included a sprinkling of normal films, since the confident appreciation of the absence of any real roentgen-based abnormalities may also be very helpful.

We would like to impress upon the nonradiologist viewer the fact that films are surveyed much more intelligently with some clinical data in mind. In training the eye, it is undoubtedly helpful to learn to survey a film first without any knowledge of the story, but a truly discriminating analysis of a film study cannot exclude the patient's presenting problem. For this reason, we have given a brief history for each patient and we have not hesitated to include some films that confirm the clinical stories and others that contradict them.

The fourth section of the book was named *The Total Patient* in the previous edition. It was based on the Massachusetts General Hospital's radiology clerkship imaging algorithm tutorials. We renamed it *Clinical Skills* to emphasize and reflect the importance of imaging skills in clinical diagnosis.

This section is divided into sequential parts designated by letters, each part adding a little more information about the patients. The parts are designed for easy thumbing by tabs. The reader should begin with any vignette in Part A and decide how he will manage the patient and what imaging methods radiology has to offer. The film studies and other clinical or imaging procedures the student "asks for" are supplied from part to part, as the story develops. Some situations are intentionally included in which radiographic studies are not needed or are actually contraindicated.

Because we feel so strongly that there can be no isolation of the roentgen investigation from the patient and his medical problems and personal concerns, we have made each case as lifelike and clinically oriented as possible.

We hope that students will enjoy being "on call" to render assistance to the patients in this book—but we hope even more that they will learn some of the ways in which radiology can be of help to them in unraveling the sometimes complex problems presented by the total patient.

Judith Korek Amorosa, M.D.

Robert A. Novelline, M.D.

Lucy Frank Squire, M.D.

Acknowledgments

The authors wish to express their gratitude to the many people who made the new edition and the original book possible: Drs. Barbara Carter, Alice Ettinger, Adele K. Friedman, Jeffery Moore and Lawrence L. Robbins; Mss. Marilyn Toth, Genevieve Cibelli, Evelyn M. DeBerardinis, Naomi Gershon, Julia Fulop and Susan Cardinale; Messrs. Thomas Ryan and Brian Lewis.

In the bone section, our admiration for Dr. Colaice's writing has prevented our making many changes. We thank Drs. Jack Edeiken, Philip Hodes, Deborah Forrester, Howard Marcus, Robert Stephens, Elbert H. Magoon and Steel Belok for their contributions to the bone section. Drs. Juan Taveras, Robert Grugan, Abel Moreyra, Theodore Stahl, John L. Nosher and members of the Radiology Group of New Brunswick have encouraged us and contributed to the clinical skills section.

Several medical students from SUNY Brooklyn, Robert Wood Johnson (RWJ) Medical School and Harvard Medical School have been helpful in evaluation of teaching material. Criticism and suggestions would be welcome for future editions or volumes.

We thank Judith Buttenbaum (RWJ) for photographing many of the cases in the clinical skills section and some in the section on the abdomen. We also wish to acknowledge Jeffrey Kaladas, Atefeh Gupta and Paula Sharkey.

We are grateful to our department chairmen who have supported our educational activities: John L. Nosher, M.D., Robert Wood Johnson University Hospital; James H. Thrall, M.D., Massachusetts General Hospital; and Joshua A. Becker, M.D., State University Hospital and Kings County Hospital.

Closest family members and friends have been very understanding during the times of preparation: Gordon, Louis, Val, Dom, Judy, Louie, Nardine, Jim, Jenny and Meredith.

Contents

1 | Chest

Introduction

Teaching is only guidance toward the excitement of discovery. The problems on the first few page spreads are a review and an amplification of the basic roentgen concepts covered in Chapter 1 of *Fundamentals of Radiology* (LFS). Without the logical habits of mind described there you cannot expect to analyze film studies systematically, nor can you anticipate your own capacity for thinking three-dimensionally about roentgen shadows.

REMEMBER THREE THINGS:

1. Roentgen white-gray-black values are the result of variations in the number of rays that have passed through the object radiographed to blacken the film. They are, therefore, *always* summation shadowgrams of all the masses in the full thickness of the object that has been interposed between beam source and film.

2. The margin of *any* shadow on the film represents a tangentially seen interface between two masses of different roentgen density (average atomic number determines roentgen density). If one of the two masses changes so that they are alike in density, there will be no differential interface and the shadow margin will disappear.

3. Awareness of the range of atomic numbers (roentgen densities) of objects or tissues plus the information you will deduce about their thickness, shape, and form *may* make it possible for you to identify an object by name from its radiograph.

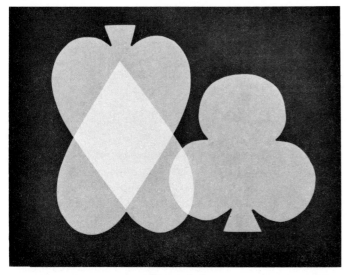

Figure 1–1

Problems

Figure 1–1. Is there a diamond in this hand?

Items to decide: Interpret the film as a summation shadowgram. What was the probable composition of the objects interposed between beam source and film? Shape? Thickness? Uniform or varied? Deduce the three-dimensional form and name/identity of the objects radiographed.

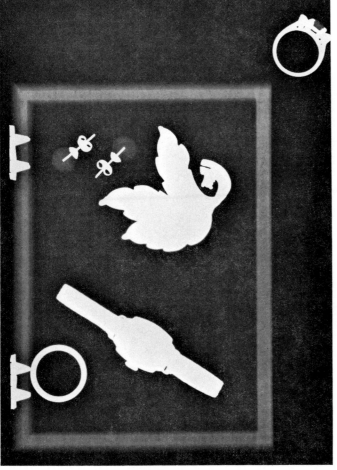

Figure 1–2

Figure 1–2. Account for the shape and form (and if possible identity) of every part of the objects radiographed. Why do the shadows of the objects have margins?

Short cut: Start by allowing intuition to suggest identity and then subject the guess you have made to logical analysis.

Answers

Figure 1–1. There is no diamond present; overlap or "summation" alone accounts for the diamond-shaped, denser area where the pointed ends of the heart and spade have been intentionally superimposed. An ellipse of the same density as that of the "diamond" is accounted for by overlap of parts of the heart and club. From their roentgen shadows you should be able to state with confidence that the three "objects" were thin, metal, of uniform thickness, cut into the shapes of heart, club, and spade and radiographed in air. (They were aluminum bridge coasters 3 mm thick.) Summate or overlap them differently and they appear as in Figure 1–3. Would they disappear if radiographed immersed in a medium composed of minute spherical granules of the same metal in a layer just 3 mm thick? (Answer on opposite page.)

Figure 1–2. This figure shows a jewel box made of wood with a hinged lid that was closed. The box contained a ring, a brooch, and a pair of (false) pearl earrings for pierced ears. A watch had been laid on top of the box. The ring outside the box had a central diamond, of good quality, at least according to its owner . . . but isn't diamond just compressed carbon? Glass filmed in air should x-ray like this, by the way, but (depending on its mineral content) may have nearly the same density as muscle in which it is embedded after injury.

In the space between the images of the watch and the brooch, summate what is actually being radiographed. (Answer on opposite page.)

The margin of any radiographic shadow is produced by a sudden change in the number of rays traversing matter or, in other words, by the existence of a tangentially seen *interface* of some sort between masses of different roentgen density, here metal and air, or wood and air. Think in terms of summation shadows and of interfaces across which x-rays slide tangentially, and you will be able to "account" for any radiographic shadow.

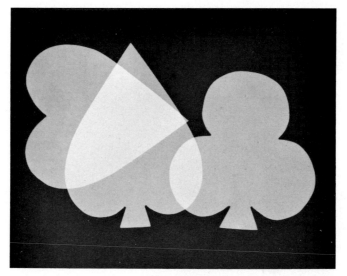

Figure 1–3

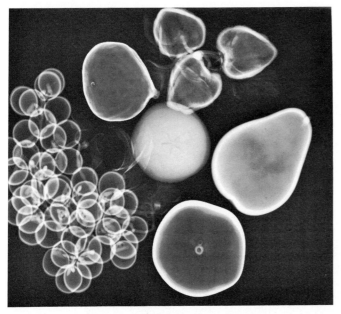

Figure 1–4

Problems

Figure 1–4. Real or artificial fruit? Why? (Analyze each roentgen shadow as a composite shadowgram with interfaces.)

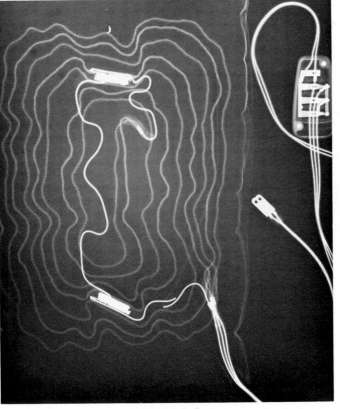

Figure 1–5

Figure 1–5. Name/identify the object radiographed. Justify your conclusion according to the basic principles roentgen shadows obey. By the way, is it "normal" or "sick"?

ANSWERS TO QUESTIONS ON PAGE 4
1. The bridge coasters would be seen faintly.
2. Top and bottom of box plus air above box and air inside box are being radiographed.

Answers

Figure 1–4. All fruit was artificial except the central piece, which was an excellent pear. The water-dense meat does not have a different density from the tough skin; the edges are more "radiolucent" because there is less pear there and more rays passed through to blacken the film. The stem is not quite perfectly superimposed on the stellate core and is seen to the left* of it as an extra dense (white) spot because it was *added* to the density of the full thickness of the pear.

The artificial fruit is seen to be hollow, the tangentially filmed shell of each accounting for the ring-like shadow, air within and air without to give you *two* air/plastic interfaces. (What would a real bunch of grapes look like if radiographed? Figure 1–6 is a radiograph of real grapes.)

Figure 1–5. A "sick" electric heating pad. It has a fractured wire. There appear to be two sorts of wires because . . . ? (Answer on Page 7.)

*The "patient's" left, remember.

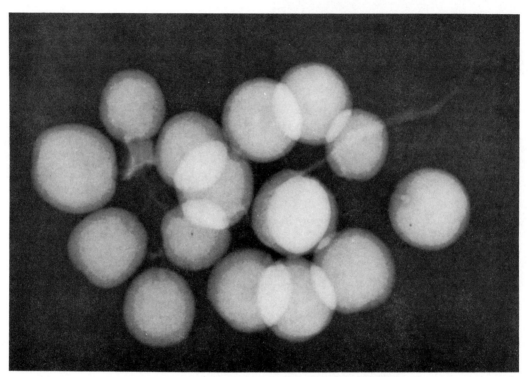

Figure 1–6 Radiograph of a bunch of real grapes.

Problems

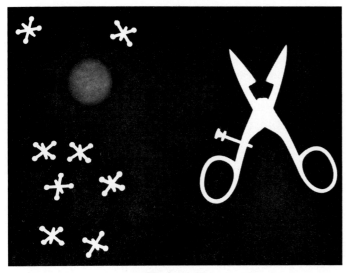

Figure 1-7

Figure 1-7. Can you name/identify the objects that have been radiographed? (Be precise—what *kind* of scissors?)

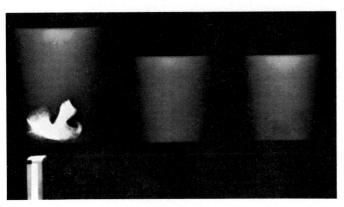

Figure 1-8

Figure 1-8. Paper cups partly filled with water, each containing a block of tissue, were radiographed from the side. What kind of tissue was immersed in water in each cup? Justify all interfaces. (The cups themselves cast no roentgen shadow.)

ADDITIONAL PROBLEMS

Predict precisely (or diagram) the radiograph of a three-inch thick slab of Swiss cheese.

Predict the appearance of a radiograph of a still-born infant.

ANSWERS CONTINUED FROM PRECEDING PAGE:

More on heating pad: *There are two sorts of electric wires in a heating pad—one a heavy copper wire of large caliber and low resistance and others that are spirals of very fine wire with a high resistance. On the original print the fine spirals could be seen clearly.*

Answers

Figure 1–7. A rubber ball, a set of jacks, and a pair of buttonhole scissors. (The screw in the handle governs the size of the hole cut.) If you failed to identify the scissors, it was probably because you did not know they existed. Neither did we. You cannot expect to identify the radiographic image of an object you have no knowledge of, nor can you be expected to figure out the changes in the radiographic appearance of tissues and structures in disease unless you are familiar with the pathology and know how it affects those tissues. (Incidentally, the vital importance of being familiar with objects, form, tissues, and pathologic change is well illustrated by the fact that we showed this radiograph to a three-year-old who had watched his mother sewing but had not played with older children. His instant response was, "That is a pair of buttonhole scissors and these are a moon and some stars." All a question of familiarity!)

Figure 1–8. Chunks of bone, fat, and muscle had been immersed in the water. The bone/water and fat/water interfaces are easy to recognize. The muscle in the center cup is the same density as the water and there is, therefore, no differential interface to outline it. (The fat did not float because it was stuck to the bottom of the cup by the time we got back to the x-ray department.)

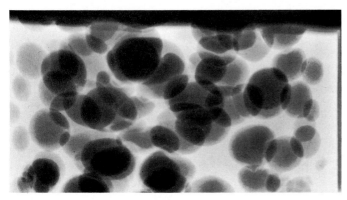

Figure 1–9

Figure 1–9: Swiss Cheese. You probably came close if you decided to think first of the *structure* radiographed—a homogeneous matrix of water density containing many empty spherical spaces, some of which would overlap others above or below and so produce elliptical areas where more rays would pass through to blacken the film.

Contrast these with the ellipses in Figure 1–6. (Incidentally, a New York taxi driver, given a little briefing in basic radiology, was able to predict the appearance of this film two hours before it was made.)

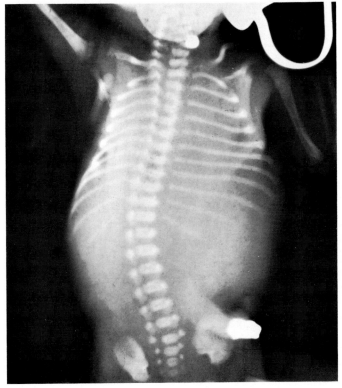

Figure 1–10

Stillborn. Stillborns, if they have never expanded their lungs or swallowed air, must be homogeneously water dense from chin to symphysis pubis. Heart, lungs, liver, spleen, and collapsed gut all have the same roentgen density and cast a confluent shadow with no boundary interfaces to outline any of these structures. The slight variations in density over the chest are skin folds. The white object over the abdomen is a metal clamp on the umbilical cord.

Read Carefully

From this point on, double page spreads with lettered *problem films,* questions relating to them, and so forth will alternate with *Answer* page spreads throughout the book. Because we think the student learns more when he has several similar film studies to look at together, each *Problem* page spread will have several films and a number of problems. You should study all the films on the page at once *before* turning to the *Answer* page spread. Use the corresponding parts and structures of all films on the same page as normals to check what you feel to be abnormal on one film. Be sure that you have thought through the answer to every question and problem on a *Problem* page spread before turning to the answers, since frequently the problems will be interrelated. One problem may help you with another on the same page. It is anticipated, however, that you will have studied the first ten chapters in *Fundamentals of Radiology* before going beyond this point. The self-checking/self-testing procedure for which the workbook is designed will be greatly enhanced and rendered much more interesting to you if you treat each new *Problem* page spread as a group of films on your own patients about which you must reach a decision, unassisted.

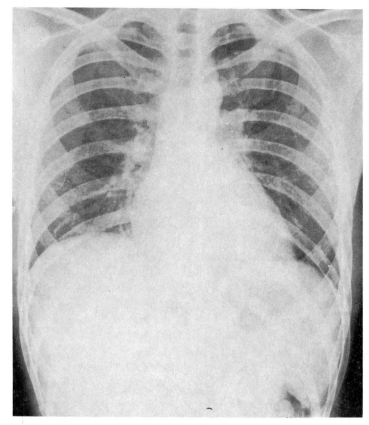

Figure 1–11   A

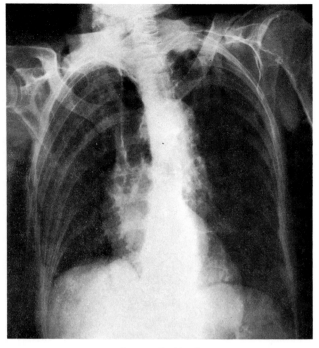

Figure 1–12   B

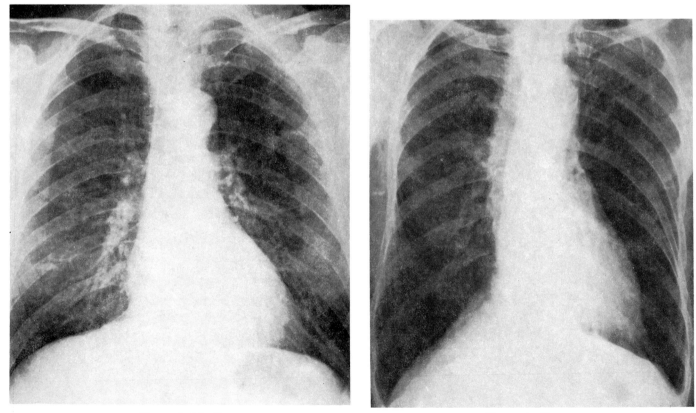

Figure 1–14   D

Figure 1–15   E

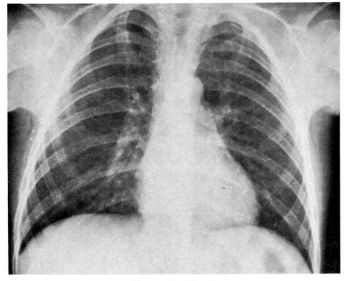

Figure 1–13 C

Problems

STUDY THESE SIX CHEST FILMS SYSTEMATICALLY

Begin with the six pairs of *clavicles*.

Are any of these films made with a *not perfect sagittal beam?*

Do any of the *hearts* appear to be enlarged?

Make a decision about each of the 12 *hemidiaphragm/lung interfaces.*

Identify three undesirable *technical imperfections.* How could the technician have avoided them? Were any justifiable, perhaps, in view of the abnormal film findings?

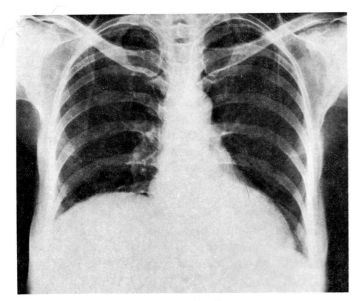

Figure 1–16 F

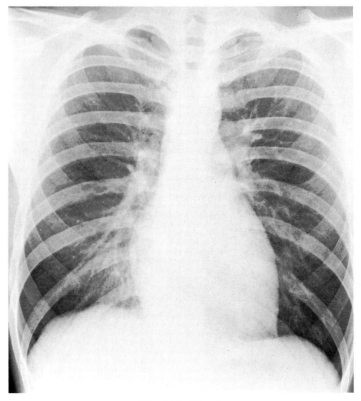

Figure 1–17   A

Answers

Clavicles are normal in **A, E,** and **F** but asymmetrical in **B,** which indicates that the patient was rotated off the sagittal plane. **D** shows a fresh fracture of the left clavicle with overriding. **C** has no clavicles, or at least only fragmentary ribbons of bone where they should be, a congenital defect.

All except **B** are made with a perfectly *sagittal beam.* Note how precisely the medial ends of the clavicles center on the white teardrop representing the spinous process of T3 in **F.** The patient in **B** was an elderly woman unable to stand and radiographed with great difficulty in her bed. Because of rotation and projection, her heart appears enlarged and her mediastinum widened.

Diaphragmatic interfaces are seen at expiration in **A;** they are normal in **B, C,** and **D** and are low, flat, and fixed at fluoroscopy in **E,** an old gentleman who had emphysema clinically. The high right diaphragm in **F** was due to a very large liver full of metastases from a carcinoma of the colon. (Note Figure 1–19, the related lateral.)

Hearts. A's heart might appear to be borderline enlarged, but the diaphragms are high (rib 9) and this is therefore a poor inspiration film. Figure 1–17 is a film made on the same patient with a good inspiration.

Technical Imperfections. A, made at expiration, was repeated at inspiration. **B** is overexposed and was not made with a sagittal beam, but the lung fields appeared clear of important pneumonic change when the film was bright-lighted, and since the patient was in great pain from a ureteral calculus, repetition of the film was felt to be unnecessary by both internist and radiologist. **A, B, D, E,** and **F** all show scapulae overlying the upper lung field, which may usually be avoided by rotating the shoulders forward. In none of these patients was it thought to be important enough to warrant repeating the film. In Patient **D,** it could not have been done anyway because of pain in the fractured clavicle.

THE LATERAL CHEST FILM

Most people find the lateral chest film a difficult muddle. There is no need to if you approach it systematically. Start with the *two diaphragmatic outlines*. The right usually appears as a clean sharp interface (lung/liver) extending from the low, pointed posterior sulcus straight forward to the anterior chest wall. The left extends forward only to the back of the cardiac shadow where the heart sits on the anterior part of the left diaphragm. The interface disappears from this point forward because the roentgen density of the left lobe of the liver and of the heart is the same.

Make a systematic visual inspection of the *two posterior sulci*, almost but not exactly superimposed in Figure 1–18. In Figure 1–19 the right is much higher than the left because of the large liver beneath the diaphragm.

Now look at the thoracic vertebrae from top to bottom. Check the density of the vertebrae on every lateral chest film since ill-defined densities in the posterior part of either lung will increase the whiteness of the vertebrae, a simple summation like that of the big liver in Figure 1–19.

The shadow of the *heart* is well anterior in the chest. In front of the heart and behind the heart are the *anterior and posterior clear spaces,* radiolucent areas where the two lungs often touch, which should be checked because either may contain masses and so become dense.

Check the *air shadow of the trachea*. The superimposed branching *hilar vessels* lie below it.

Now that you have studied the lateral chest systematically, you should be able to "account for" that large, dense, white wedge overlying the lower part of the heart in Figure 1–19. It can be "summated" as "carcinoma-filled liver plus heart plus breast." Did you note that the patient in Figure 1–18 is male and the one in Figure 1–19 female?

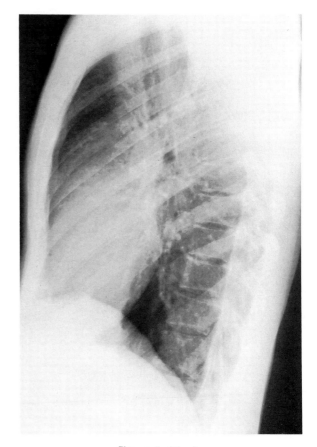

Figure 1–18 A

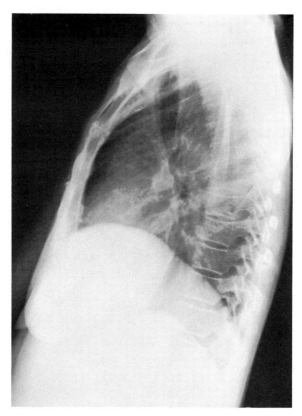

Figure 1–19 F

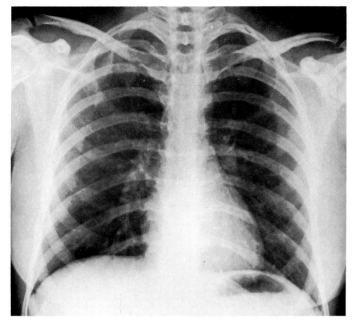

Figure 1-20 A

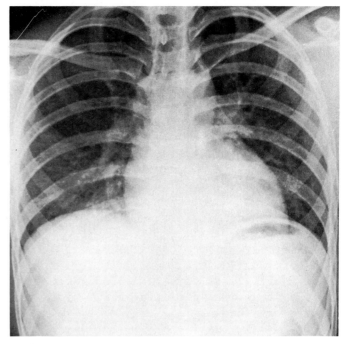

Figure 1-21 B

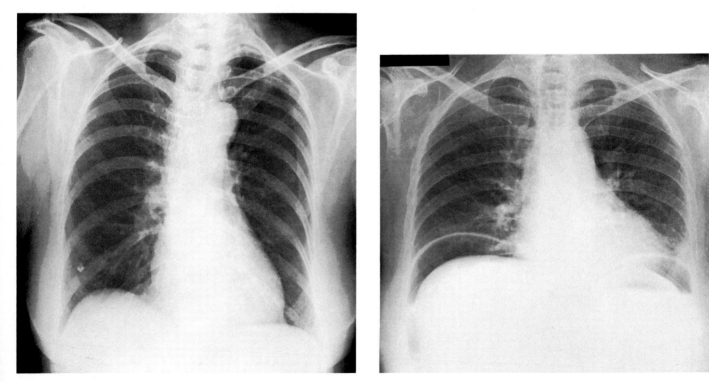

Figure 1-23 D

Figure 1-24 E

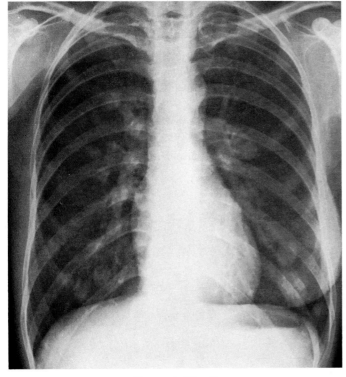

Figure 1-22   C

Problems

STUDY AND ANALYZE SYSTEMATICALLY THESE SIX PATIENTS

Which films can you be absolutely certain were taken standing?

Do you think any of these people have cardiac enlargement?

Would you have any films repeated?

How many women are there among the six?

One of these patients fell off a horse a year ago; can you figure out which one?

One of these patients had major surgery a year ago and one will have surgery this afternoon—which?

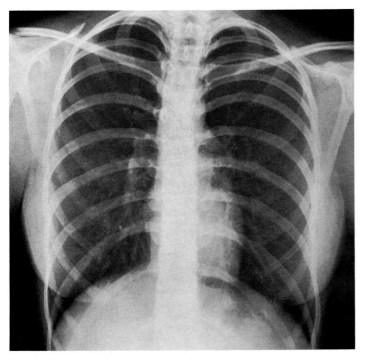

Figure 1-25   F

Answers

Patients **A, B, C,** and **E** are *standing* because there are fluid levels where the ray slides tangentially across an interface between air and gastric contents. In addition, the patient in **E** has fluid/air interfaces at both sides of the upper abdomen that are too close to the lateral abdominal wall to be intraluminal. These tell you that the patient has free air and fluid in the peritoneal space. She was a middle-aged woman sitting quietly in clinic, having had an appointment for ten days to "see about" her recurrent ulcer symptoms. Note the interface that represents the outside of the gastric fundus outlined by free air under the left diaphragm. Figure 1–26 is her lateral film.

B and **E** are poor inspiration films. *Repeat* film **B** (Fig. 1–26). There is no time and no need to repeat **E**.

All were *women* except **B**, a young man whose gastric fluid level on this occasion was a CO_2/Pepsi-Cola interface. The breasts in **E** were heavy and pendulous and hard to see on either the posteroanterior *(PA)* or the lateral view.

The woman you see in **A** actually did *fall off a horse* and has an old, well-healed fracture of her left clavicle. The patient in **D** has a calcification in the right lower lung field that proved to be in the right breast. It is faintly seen in Figure 1–27.

Surgery. The patient in **C** had a radical mastectomy a year ago and now has multiple round pulmonary metastases. Contrast the high arched soft tissue of skin fold on the right, where breast and pectoral muscles have been removed, with the gentle curve on the left, where the axillary fold joins the remaining breast. The patient in **E** had emergency surgery as soon as it could be arranged that afternoon, the perforated ulcer was repaired, and she made a good recovery.

F is a normal chest film and Figure 1–28 is that patient's lateral.

Note: The occasional interpolation of *normal films* throughout the workbook is intended to enhance your enjoyment of the exercises, and, after all, more nearly corresponds to the assortment of film problems common to your professional workday. The automatic bias with which we all approach the usual CPC exercise decreases its meaningfulness as an inducement to think sensibly.

Use page 17 as a review exercise in analyzing the lateral chest film. (But beware the garden path!)

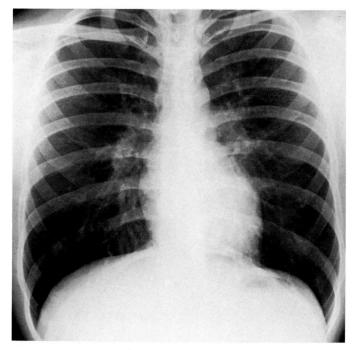

Figure 1–26   B

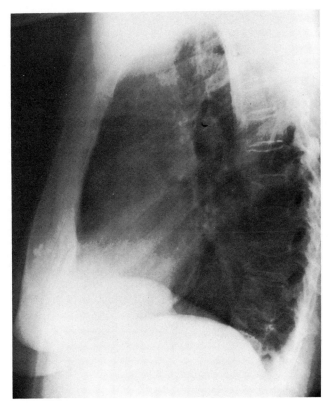

Figure 1–27   D

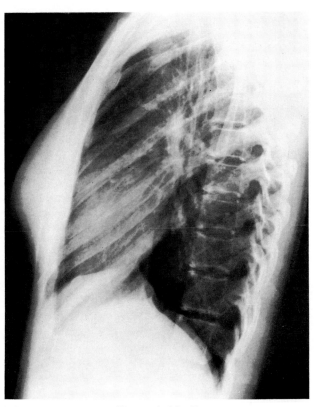

Figure 1–28   F

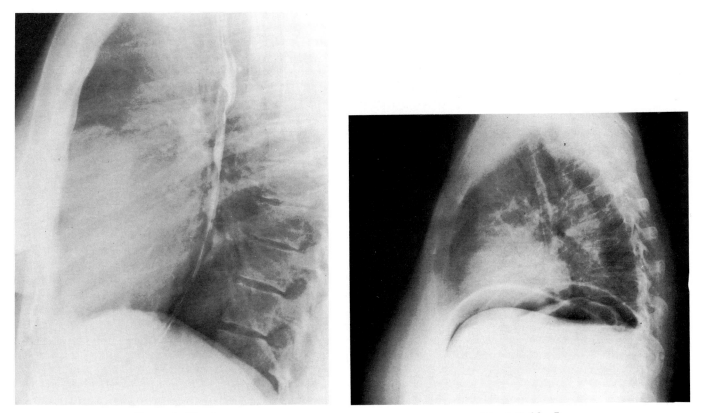

Figure 1–29   ?

Figure 1–30   E

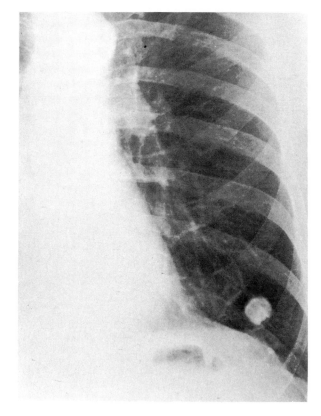

Figure 1-31   A

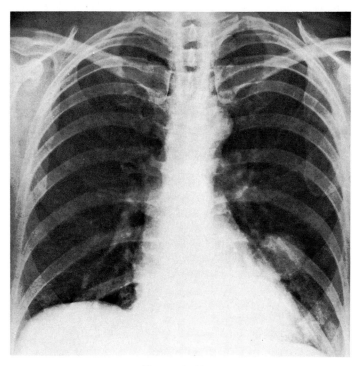

Figure 1-32   B

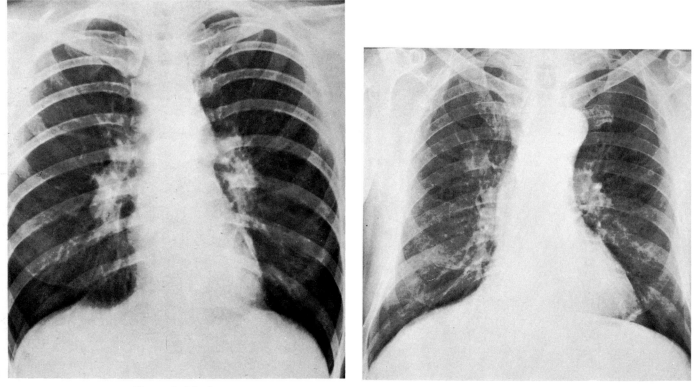

Figure 1-34   D

Figure 1-35   E

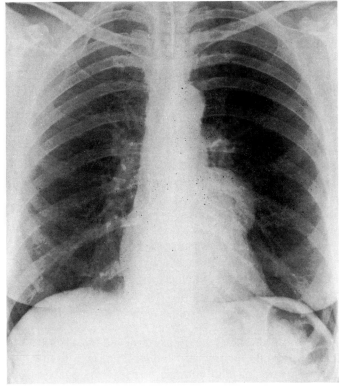

Figure 1–33   C

These six patients were entirely asymptomatic. Examine their chest films as you would if they had come to you for an annual check-up. All were within a year or so of age 40 except **E,** who was 57.

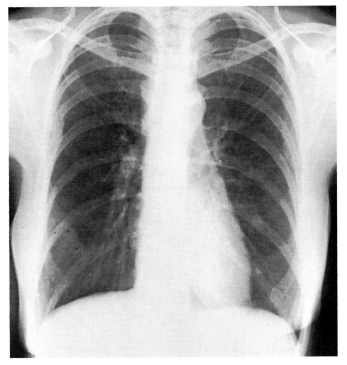

Figure 1–36   F

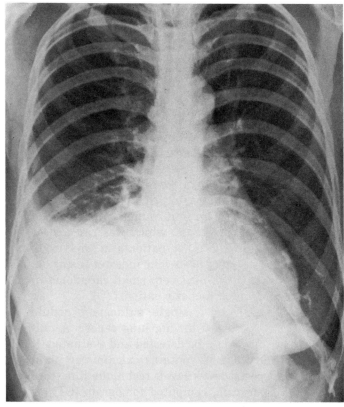

Figure 1-40   A

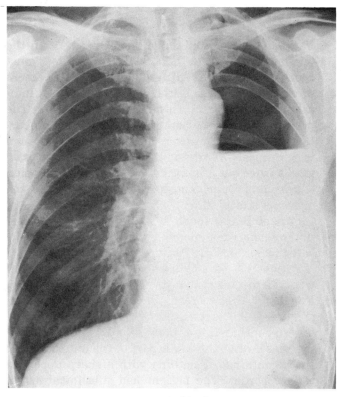

Figure 1-41   B

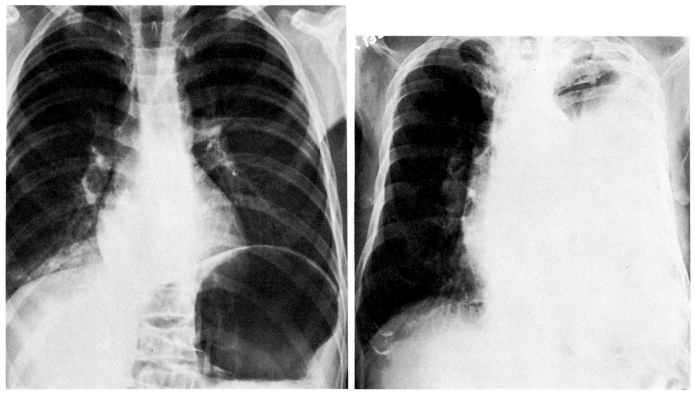

Figure 1-43   D

Figure 1-44   E

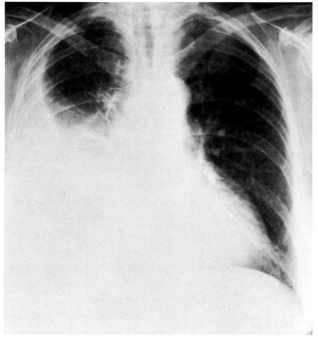

Figure 1–42 C

Problems

Check these six films for rotation and for degree of inspiration. All six patients had *dyspnea* and *chest pain*. **A** and **D** had fever. Anticipate the roentgen shadows on the lateral chest films in **A, B, C,** and **D**.

Is there a valid *mediastinal shift* in any of these films?

How many have *pleural effusion*?

Has any of these patients roentgen evidence of *previous surgery,* recent or remote?

On which would you want supplementary film studies? Anticipate the appearance of the ones you request.

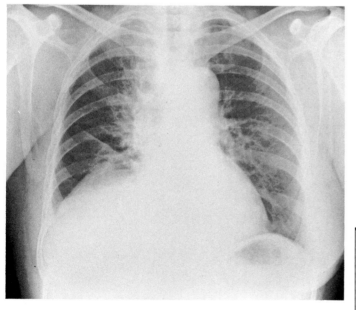

Figure 1–45 F

When studying answers place edge of page 24 in center of page 22 in order to view PA film and related lateral on the same patient together. This arrangement for viewing is set up throughout the book.

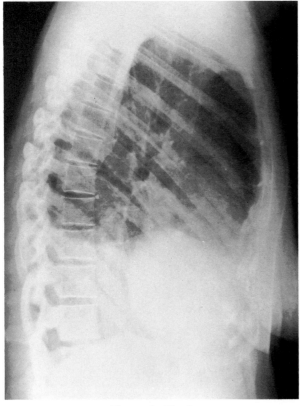

Figure 1–46　A

Answers

All the films are made with a sagittal beam; none is rotated.

All six films were made at *deep inspiration for that patient*. There is therefore no point in repeating any of these films. Note that in **A**, although the right diaphragmatic leaf is at the tenth rib, the left leaf has been pulled down almost to the twelfth. In each patient one of the two diaphragms is obscured or high, but you can estimate inspiratory effort from the other.

One would request lateral films on **A, D,** and **F,** hoping for more information about the posterior sulci and lower lung fields. In **B, C,** and **E** there is not much to be gained from a lateral film since the pleural effusion is so large that it will obscure other film findings. Figure 1–50 is the related lateral to **B.** The patient had had a left pneumonectomy a few days before and has the expected hydropneumothorax.

In **A** *some* fluid in the right sinus together with a high "diaphragm" suggests infrapulmonary fluid. Figure 1–46 shows fluid in one posterior sulcus. In the *lateral decubitus film* (Fig. 1–49) the fluid has been dumped out and lies against the lateral chest wall.

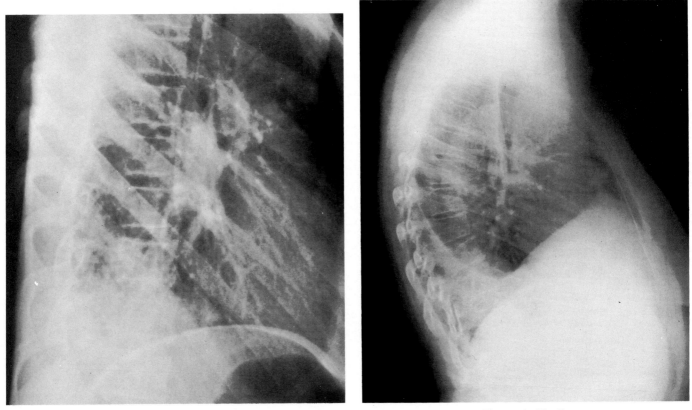

Figure 1–47　D

Figure 1–48　F

Note: The normal lower right lung may now be seen. The white triangle over the heart is a summation of heart plus breast.

Patient **D** had a right *lower lobe pneumonia*, seen near the heart and just above the diaphragm. In the lateral film (Fig. 1–47) only one diaphragm is visible, the left, outlined from both sides by air. The right diaphragmatic interface has disappeared posteriorly because of the confluence of pneumonic lung and liver shadow.

With regard to *mediastinal shift*, remember that the normal location for the trachea is in the midline down to the clavicles and then displaced slightly to the right by the arch of the aorta. In **B** it is shifted slightly *toward* the side of the effusion; the volume of the hydropneumothorax does not exactly equal the volume of the missing left lung. The normal course after pneumonectomy is for the mediastinum to shift gradually farther and farther to the side of the missing lung as air and fluid are resorbed until the pleural space is obliterated and the heart lies against the chest wall. The appearance of the chest film will then almost exactly resemble that for total collapse of one lung.

The lower trachea and right heart shadow in patient **E** *are* shifted to the right by this very large effusion. In **C, E,** and **F** the effusion was due to malignant seeding of the pleura. (What! You hadn't noticed the missing right breast in **F**?) Much of the fluid in **F** is infrapulmonary and some is probably loculated in the fissures (Fig. 1–48).

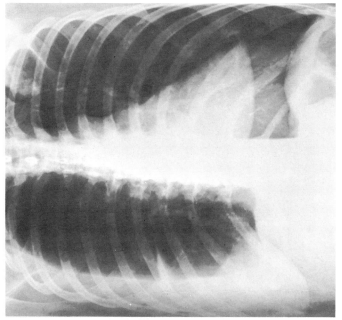

Figure 1–49 A

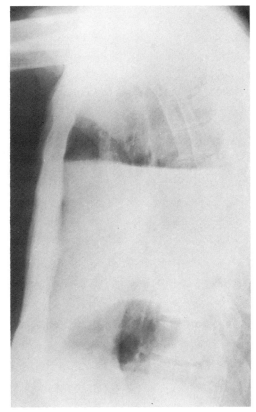

Figure 1–50 B

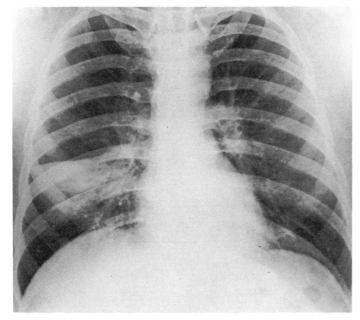

Figure 1–51   Bill Dean.

Problems

It is your evening on duty in the emergency division. You see these four patients within two hours.

Bill Dean and *Ann Pulsifer*, both under 25, complain of *chest pain, fever, and cough* for about 48 hours. Both were well a week ago. You do careful physical examinations on both patients and fill out requisitions for chest films (to include the appropriate laterals).

Mr. Dean has rales anteriorly but his posterior base is clear. He has a white count of 11,000.

Miss Pulsifer is much more toxic, has rales and dullness to percussion posteriorly, and her white count is 18,000.

From your experience on the preceding page spreads, have you any roentgen evidence here for a hydropneumothorax in either patient? Why? Why not?

If you think pneumonic consolidation could explain either of the curious "straight-line" interfaces, precisely what part of the lung would be involved? Anticipate the lateral film in each.

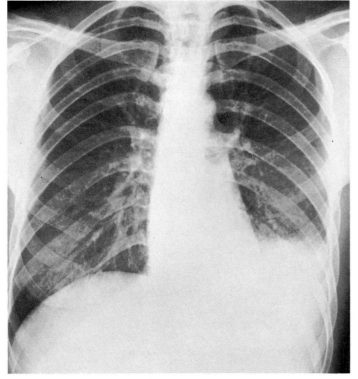

Figure 1–52   Ann Pulsifer.

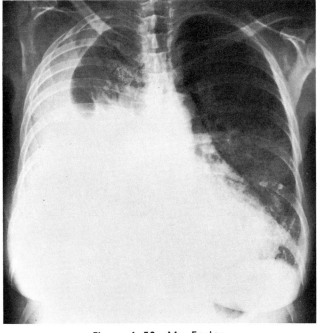

Figure 1-53 Mrs. Foster.

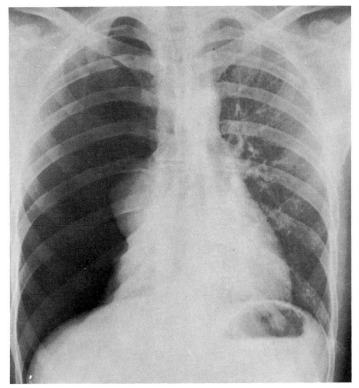

Figure 1-54 Mr. Adams.

Later you examine *Mrs. Foster* and *Mr. Adams*, who both come to the hospital because of *increasing dyspnea.*

Mrs. Foster is afebrile and had a completely negative general physical check-up four months ago.

Mr. Adams has not been seen here before and was well yesterday. He has had some chest pain for 24 hours but has no fever or cough.

What do you find in each on physical examination? Explain the dyspnea both dynamically and physiologically.

ALL NAMES ARE, OF COURSE, FICTIONAL THROUGHOUT THE BOOK.

Fold the margin of this page in to the center of the book and you will be able to examine the lateral films on Mr. Dean and Miss Pulsifer together with their PA chest films. Do the lateral films change your mind about anything you had decided?

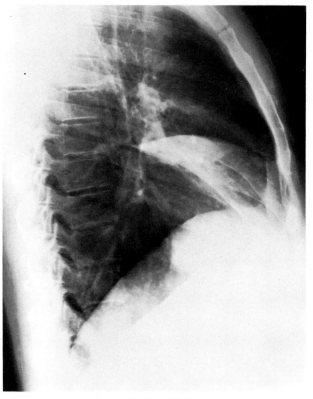

Figure 1-55 Bill Dean.

Answers

In *Mr. Dean* and *Miss Pulsifer*, neither of the "straight-line" interfaces could be a pleural fluid level. There is nothing to indicate a hydropneumothorax since normal lung markings are seen extending straight to the chest wall. There is no curving line in either patient to suggest pleural fluid.

The lateral on Mr. Dean shows you the triangular shadow across the heart that you have come to associate with middle lobe consolidation (Fig. 1-55). The horizontal interface seen in the PA chest film is between consolidated middle lobe and aerated upper lobe. The heart/lung interface in the PA view has been preserved so Mr. Dean must have pneumonia involving only the lateral segment of his middle lobe, the medial segment having been spared.

Miss Pulsifer's lost diaphragm is explained when you see the lateral (Fig. 1-56). Only one diaphragmatic interface is seen, the normal right. She has consolidation of the four basilar segments of the left lower lobe and the apical segment has been spared. The "straight line" in the PA view is the irregular top of the consolidation.

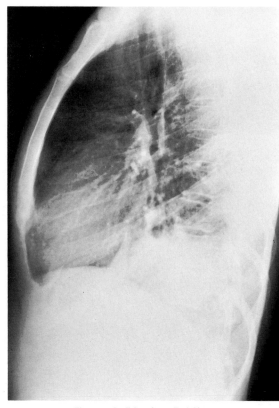

Figure 1-56 Ann Pulsifer.

In Figures 1–57 and 1–58 you have follow-up films on Miss Pulsifer. Note the reappearance of *two* diaphragmatic interfaces.

Mrs. Foster has a massive pleural effusion extending over the apex of the right lung and displacing the mediastinum to the left. Right thoracentesis showed clear fluid. Malignant cells were found on cytologic examination, metastatic from a carcinoma of the breast. A unilateral massive effusion is usually malignant in origin.

Mr. Adams has a pneumothorax with almost complete collapse of the right lung and slight shift of the mediastinum to the left, suggesting the possibility of tension pneumothorax. Of the four patients it would be Mr. Adams whom you should attend to first, of course, since tension pneumothorax can be a disaster and should be decompressed early. Predict the position of the mediastinum on inspiration/expiration films. His dyspnea was appreciably relieved by prompt removal of air from the pleural space via chest tube. Dyspnea must have been the result of decreased oxygenation with only one working lung and great reduction in the venous return to the heart with such an increase in intrathoracic pressure.

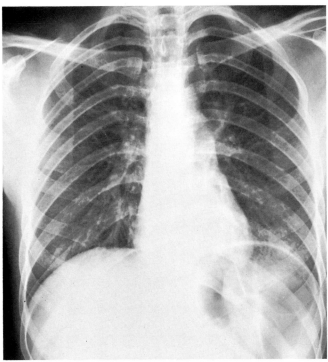

Figure 1–57 Ann Pulsifer.

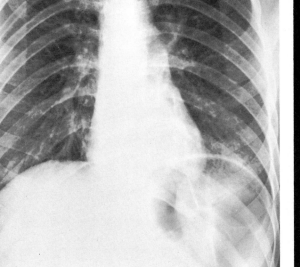

Figure 1–58 Ann Pulsifer.

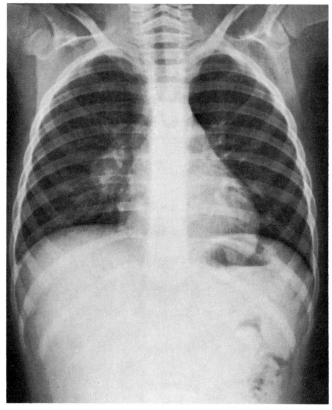

Figure 1-59   A

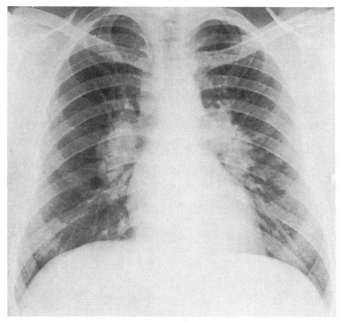

Figure 1-60   B

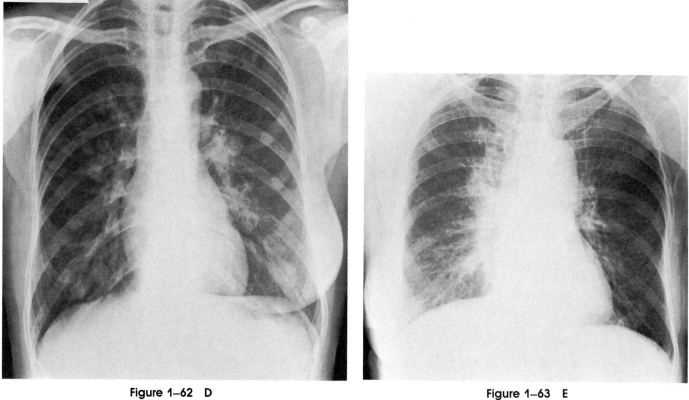

Figure 1-62   D

Figure 1-63   E

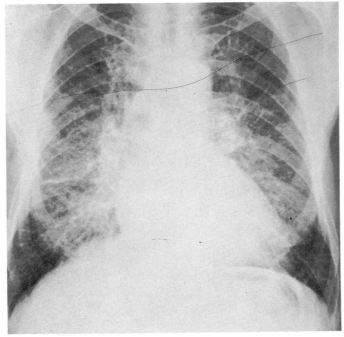

Figure 1–61   C

Problems

Are there any roentgen findings here that give you a clue as to the *age* of any of these six patients?

On physical examination one of these patients had an *enlarged spleen* but is not acutely ill. Can you pick out which one?

Two patients have nontender *cervical lymph nodes.* Which two?

Three are *dyspneic.* Which three? Why are they short of breath?

Patient **F**, acutely ill with *chest pain*, has just been admitted to the emergency division. He claims he has never been sick a day in his life before this afternoon. Patient **C** has been sick in bed at home for two months. Both have *enlarged livers*. Why do you think they are enlarged and what would you expect to find on microscopic inspection of liver tissue?

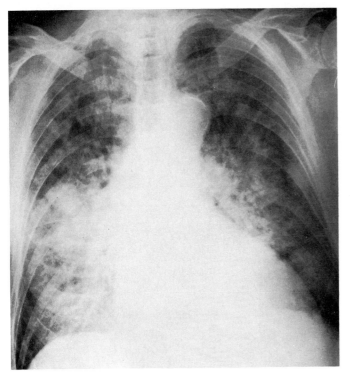

Figure 1–64   F

Answers

Age. Patient **A** is a child, evident when you discover his unfused humeral epiphyses. Mr. **F** is an older man with a large heart and heavily calcified aorta.

The *spleen* is visible and normal in the child, **A**. Patient **B** could have sarcoidosis or Hodgkin's disease. None of the other patients has findings suggesting any disease process usually associated with splenomegaly.

Both **A** and **B** had nontender *cervical nodes*. The child had glandular tuberculosis and a node in the right hilum that regressed under therapy. **B** had Hodgkin's disease (proved by node biopsy) and a big spleen. Figure 1–65 is his lateral film.

Patients **C** and **F** were *dyspneic* because of cardiac failure, acute in **F** and chronic in **C**. (Note Kerley's B lines in Figure 1–61 in the right lower lung field near the chest wall and also the extrapleural edema.) Both these patients had been hypertensive for some time and have large hearts. Figure 1–66 shows Patient **C** a year earlier.

Patient **F** had a massive myocardial infarction a few hours ago and is in acute pulmonary edema.

Mr. **C** has big engorged hila and his *large liver* would show chronic passive congestion. With Patient **F**'s brief history his large liver was harder to explain until a week or so later (Fig. 1–69) when his edema had cleared on management and the pulmonary metastases from his unsuspected colon carcinoma emerged from their surrounding fluid. At autopsy a month later his liver was almost entirely replaced with carcinoma.

Patient **D** had a right mastectomy some time ago and now has many round pulmonary metastases. She was not dyspneic.

Patient **E** had a left mastectomy two years ago and now returns complaining of steadily increasing dyspnea. She has a widened mediastinal shadow and lymphangitic spread of carcinoma outward from the mediastinum into the peribronchial lymphatics.

Figures 1–66 and 1–67, normal chest films, are supplied for comparison with all other hilar shadows.

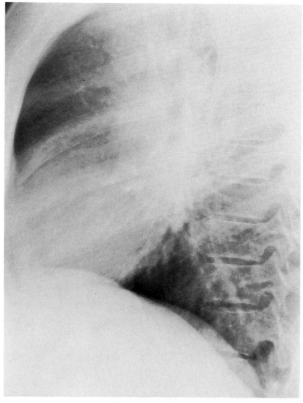

Figure 1–65   B

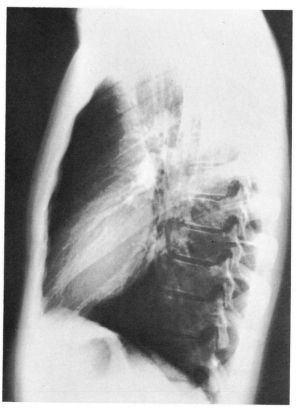

Figure 1–66   Normal.

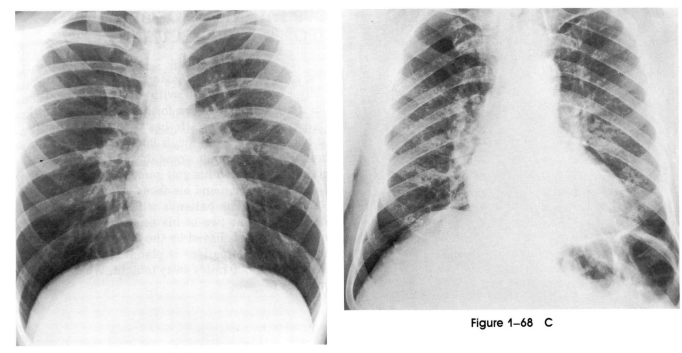

Figure 1-67 Normal.

Figure 1-68 C

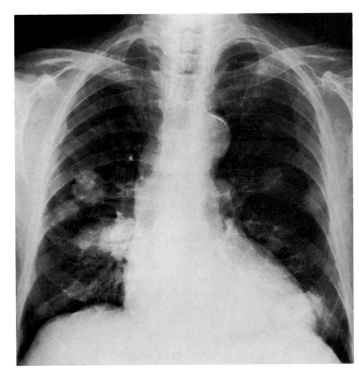

Figure 1-69 F

. . . BUT NONE OF WHOM HAVE IT

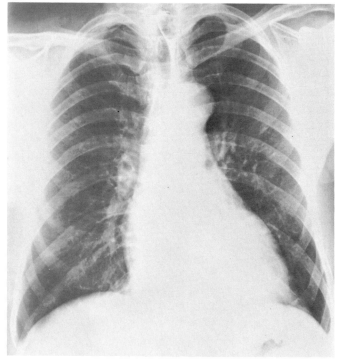

Figure 1–74 Mr. D. B.

Mr. Dupuy-Bambleschnitzler has a large heart, engorged hila, and increased vascular pulmonary markings. He is in early-to-moderate congestive heart failure. You persuade him to send his second-in-command (or Mrs. D. B.) to the sales meeting and admit him to the hospital after treatment for congestive heart failure. Figure 1–74 is his follow-up film. (He has nothing to suggest pulmonary tuberculosis.)

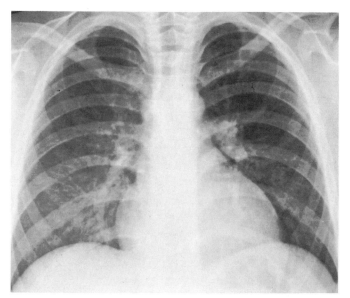

Figure 1–75 Tommy P.

Tommy has a diffusely disseminated bronchopneumonia, more advanced on the right. Streptococci were obtained from his sputum. The film findings alone might just possibly be those of a fulminant pulmonary acid-fast infection in a child, but neither the very acute picture clinically nor the rapid recovery was consistent with tuberculosis. He recovered on antibiotics within a week. Figure 1–75 is his PA film a week later. Figures 1–76 and 1–77 are his early and late lateral films.

(If you fold in the page margin you can look at all four films together.)

Mr. Flashman has a markedly widened mediastinal shadow and a right pleural effusion. The mass is confluent with the heart shadow and probably applied closely against it. The differential possibilities include all the anterior mediastinal masses that may be found in young adults. Of these, lymphoma is the most likely in this patient. The possibility of tuberculosis, in spite of the history, is remote. Thoracentesis produced a clear, sterile fluid with no cells; it was probably, therefore, a mechanical transudate. Node biopsy showed lymphoma.

Mr. Spinelli's striking weight loss must be explained. His film shows a widened mediastinum and his physical findings suggest tracheal compression. (An overexposed film or a tomogram would have shown this better.) With this picture, the first consideration for a patient in his age group must be bronchogenic carcinoma with mediastinal metastases encasing the trachea and major bronchi. Often other structures are also involved, such as the superior vena cava, the esophagus, and the recurrent laryngeal or phrenic nerves. With a history of a normal chest film four months ago, his strikingly abnormal film findings are strong presumptive evidence for new growth rather than any sort of tuberculous involvement in spite of the history. Biopsy was taken of a supraclavicular node and radiation therapy started, but the patient died suddenly a week after this film was made. At autopsy he was found to have extensive early mediastinal spread from a dime-sized carcinoma in the right main stem bronchus. Bronchoscopic study had been unsatisfactory because of the tracheal narrowing to less than half its normal dimension.

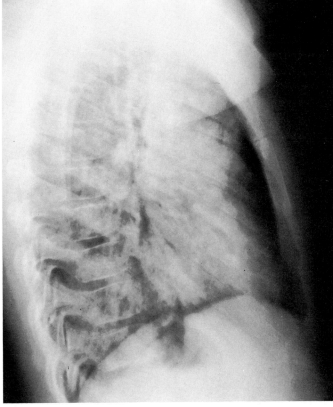

Figure 1–76   Tommy P.

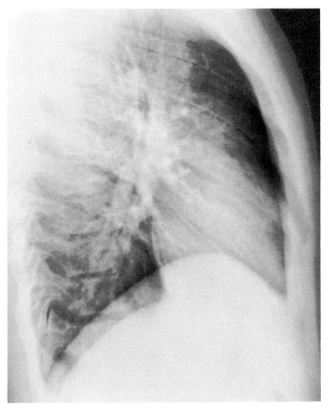

Figure 1–77   Tommy P.

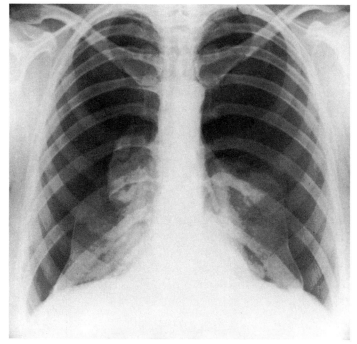

Figure 1–78 A
(Mrs. Pardiggle).

Problems

Explain *shortness of breath* in each of these five patients. (Note that Figures 1–79 and 1–84 are of one patient and Figures 1–80 and 1–81 are of one patient.) All were extremely ill; **C** and **E** had high fevers; the rest were afebrile.

Which have the bleakest prognoses?

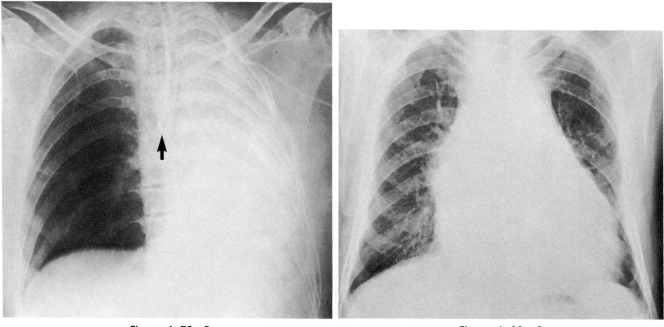

Figure 1–79 B
(Harold Skimpole).

Figure 1–80 C
(Mr. Snagsby).

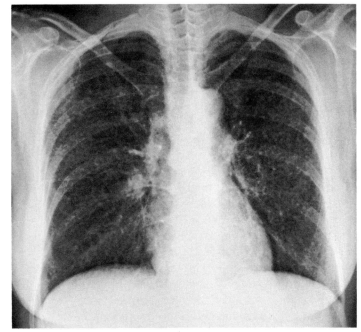

Figure 1–82   D
(Volumnia Deadlock).

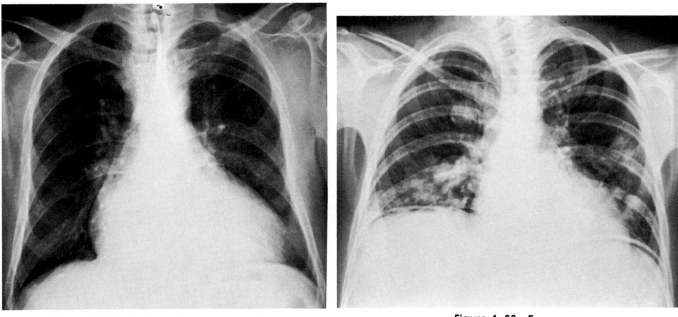

Figure 1–81   Mr. Snagsby, a year earlier.

Figure 1–83   E
(Mr. Tulkingham).

Answers

A, *Mrs. Pardiggle*, had sudden chest pain two hours ago while cleaning her basement and has been dyspneic at rest ever since. She has a bilateral 60 to 75 per cent pneumothorax (Fig. 1–78). No lung markings are seen beyond the margins of the collapsing lungs. The white line bordering the lungs is visceral pleura seen tangentially. Note how the heart/lung interfaces are disappearing as the roentgen density of the lung approaches that of heart muscle. Mrs. Pardiggle had had two previous episodes of spontaneous pneumothorax; she probably ruptured emphysematous blebs during her housecleaning exertions. Her dyspnea was, of course, the result of sudden decrease in functioning lung tissue and was present even as she lay quietly in bed.

This is an example of collapse of lung due to compression from air in the pleural space.

B, *Mr. Skimpole*, has a collapsed left lung but no pneumothorax to push it in against the mediastinum. This is a straight sagittal film and, therefore, there is a valid and marked displacement of the mediastinum to the left. The density occupying the left hemithorax is, then, the heart and great vessels, together with the airless left lung lying against the chest wall. Dyspnea is due to sudden decrease in functioning lung tissue.

Now note that the endotracheal tube is in the *right* main bronchus. The film was made because the patient, postoperative after an emergency appendectomy with general anesthesia, rapidly became cyanotic and tachypneic in the recovery room. When the tube was withdrawn well above the carina and suction applied, the left lung re-expanded quite readily. (Figure 1–84 was made two hours after Figure 1–79.)

Here collapse is of a quite different character and the airlessness of the lung is due to bronchial obstruction and secondary resorption of air.

C, *Mr. Snagsby* (Fig. 1–80), has marked cardiomegaly and a missing left sixth rib. He had surgery to a stenosed aortic valve two years ago. Figure 1–81 is a film made a year ago, before his present illness. Note the difference in the width of the mediastinum. He was admitted with substernal pain and a temperature of 40.6° C. He was delirious and extremely restless. Surgical decompression of the mediastinum revealed a large mediastinal abscess. This was drained and the patient put on high doses of antibiotics. After a stormy period of recovery an additional complaint of dysphagia could be investigated by barium swallow, and an esophageal carcinoma was found that had perforated into the mediastinum. His dyspnea was due to mechanical compression of the trachea and bronchi from edema and exudate under pressure.

D, *Mrs. Deadlock*, had an occupational history of having worked (for six months only and that 20 years ago) in a tubular illumination plant making fluorescent light bulbs. Her dyspnea has been gradually increasing and her chest film shows the myriad small disseminated shadows throughout both lungs seen in injury to the lung from beryllium (Fig. 1–82). These represent the shadows of granulomas and scar tissue, and they are less striking on the chest film than microscopically because of the "subtraction effect" of the marked accompanying emphysema. The dyspnea is explained by the extensive parenchymal changes and associated thickening of the alveolar walls that cause "alveolar-capillary block" and interference with the exchange of gases.

E, *Mr. Tulkingham*, has high diaphragms with air under both and multiple round densities in the lungs. He had a bilateral adrenal ablation a year ago for adrenal carcinoma and has been on maintenance hormone management. This was directly related to the perforation of his gastric ulcer four days ago. At the time this film was made he had peritonitis and high, fixed diaphragms (Fig. 1–83). His dyspnea was due to pain, limited diaphragmatic motion, and small tidal air.

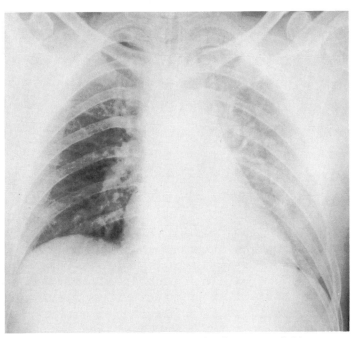

Figure 1–84 Mr. Skimpole, later the same night.

The curious names? All characters in Dickens' *Bleak House*. **C**, **D**, and **E** had very bleak prognoses, but **A** and **B** recovered promptly.

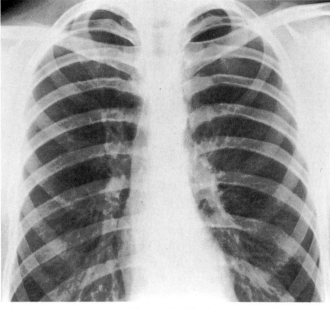

Figure 1–85 A

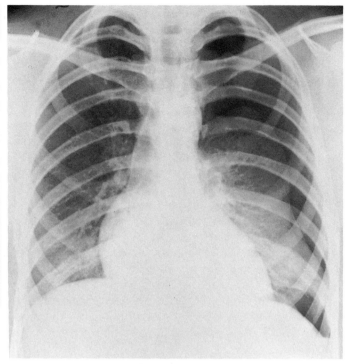

Figure 1–86 B

Problems

Patient **A** (Fig. 1–85) had slight chest pain an hour ago. Study the film, comparing carefully the markings in bilaterally symmetrical interspaces.

Now perhaps you have recognized the margin of partially collapsed left lung and the presence of pneumothorax on that side. The air imprisoned in the pleural space is a trifle more radiolucent than blood-perfused lung even at inspiration. At expiration this "cushion of air" is compressed.

Now study **B** (Fig. 1–86), an expiration film made on the same patient. There the difference in density between pneumothorax and partially collapsed left lung is much greater, and there is a striking contrast between the density of the two lungs, something which was not evident at once even on the original film for **A**. The implication is clear—we know that both lungs are less radiolucent at expiration than when fully expanded, and here in **B** one

is contrasting *three* different densities: normal right lung at expiration, partially collapsed left lung also at expiration, and free air in the pleural space. The *difference* between the latter two is greater at expiration than it is at inspiration, and the expiration film is therefore much more likely to show the presence of a small pneumothorax that might otherwise escape our notice. Perhaps it would be well to order such a series routinely in patients with sudden chest pain.

Note, too, the short horizontal fluid/air interface in the left costophrenic sinus, another clue to the presence of pneumothorax. The mediastinum appears to bow to the right on both films. Now study **C** and **D** and **E** and **F** (Figs. 1–87 to 1–90), two more pairs of inspiration-expiration films. Both patients had had chest pain of two hours' duration, but were perfectly well that morning. (Be sure to decide about mediastinal shift.)

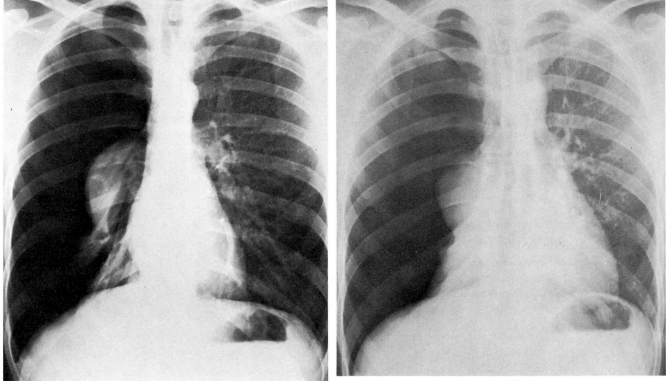

Figure 1–87   C

Figure 1–88   D

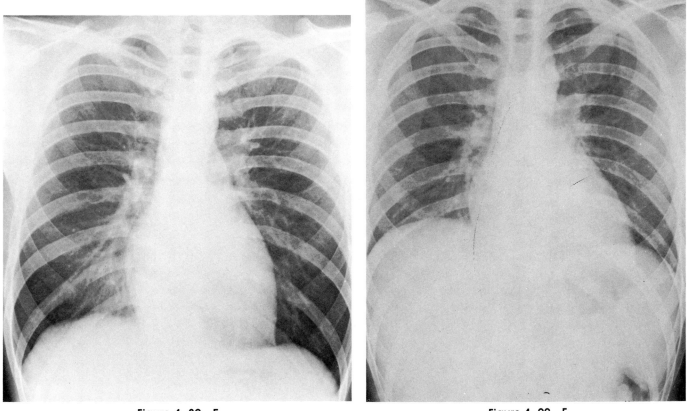

Figure 1–89   E

Figure 1–90   F

Answers

Patient **C–D** has a large right pneumothorax and almost total collapse of the right lung with rather pronounced mediastinal shift to the left on expiration. The picture raises the question of a tension pneumothorax. Note how the trapped pleural air seems to bulge into the left hemithorax across the heart shadow in **D**. After chest tube placement there was a dramatic release of air.

E and **F** are normal chest films at inspiration and expiration. The patient was apparently having an acute gallbladder attack and possibly passing a stone. He subsequently localized his pain to the upper abdomen and back and was transiently jaundiced. **F** was made first, rejected because of the poor inspiration, and then **E** was obtained.

If you called **E** a normal chest film, be sure to recognize with relief and encouragement your own progress in discrimination and judgment about roentgen findings. Remember, it is always a normal chest film until you can find something definitely wrong with it.

Review Quiz

The films on this page spread were *all* made on patients with *chest pain of a few hours' duration*, so you have another chance to differentiate between valid roentgen findings and others that must be discounted for one reason or another. All these patients were in the hospital for at least one night.

(Study in *lettered* order. Answers on page 47.)

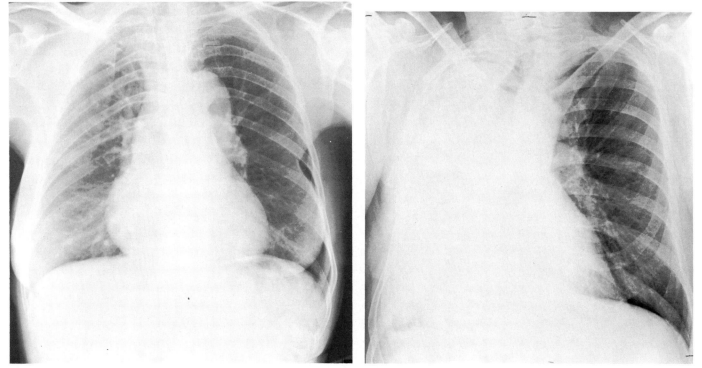

Figure 1–91 A   Figure 1–92 B

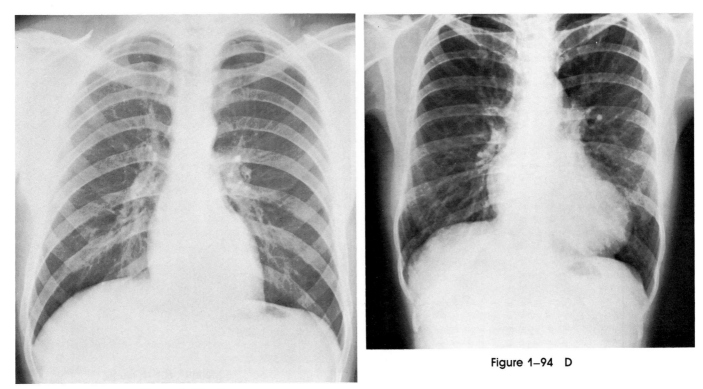

Figure 1-93   C

Figure 1-94   D

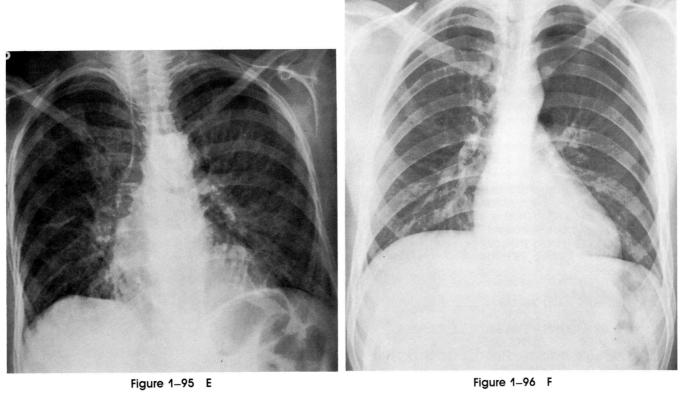

Figure 1-95   E

Figure 1-96   F

Answers to Problems on Pages 44 and 45

A shows a fair degree of rotation, but *is* the heart really enlarged? Figure 1–104 is a film made on the same patient with a straight sagittal beam. Chest pain in this patient proved to be due to angina. She was hypertensive and the heart is larger than normal.

There is also slight rotation in Figure 1–95, but Mr. **E** was very ill, very dyspneic, very anxious, and in a good deal of pain. He was in acute left heart failure, the result of a myocardial infarction of several hours' duration. He was very hard to position, and you have definite roentgen signs here and need not repeat the film.

There is no rotation in young Mr. **C**. His rather small, spontaneous pneumothorax on the left could be seen in retrospect on the original film but had been missed until an expiration film (**F**) was made. You can now see the lateral margin of the left lung. The upper mediastinum is not shifted, although the heart tilts to the left on expiration. Recovery was prompt.

Patient **D**, with no rotation and diaphragms fairly well down, has exaggerated and somewhat tortuous vascular markings throughout both lungs (compare the same parts of each lung with **C** beside it). The cardiac shadow is generous and *appears* to show left ventricular prominence. This is not an infrequent illusion when there is *right* ventricular hypertrophy, here due to interatrial septal defect, a left-to-right shunt, and recirculation of 30 per cent of blood returned from the lungs. The patient had had a characteristic murmur since childhood, and the slightly elevated cardiac apex tipped up away from the diaphragm was correctly interpreted as displacement of a normal left ventricle by the enlarged right ventricle. The same appearance characterizes the coeur en sabot seen in tetralogy, for the same reason. It is well to remember that we cannot evaluate left ventricular size with certainty from the PA radiograph in the presence of right ventricular enlargement. Sometimes lateral films help: the left ventricle enlarges downward and posteriorly in this view while the right ventricle fills in the retrosternal space.

Chest pain in this patient was esophageal and was due to a poorly chewed piece of meat lodged near the cardia. The pain was relieved when the meat passed through into the stomach.

The patient shown in **B** must have either a collapsed or an absent right lung. The left diaphragm is below the tenth rib and the clavicles are symmetrical in appearance; therefore, the strikingly shifted position of the trachea must be a valid finding. Lung collapse should be your first thought if you are sure the patient has not had a pneumonectomy. This one had. The chest pain proved to be due to recurrence of the lung cancer.

Answers to Problems on Pages 46 and 47

If your filled-in answers are correct, you have a vertical acrostic reading "I'M NO FOOL." Congratulations on both counts!

Patient **L** has a right middle lobe (RML) consolidation with no decrease in size of the lobe (lateral view). The right heart/lung interface has been lost. The mediastinum is not shifted. In the PA view you are seeing the vessels for the lower lobe superimposed on homogeneously dense middle lobe.

Patient **N** had an RML pneumonia clinically, too, but her middle lobe is decreased in size as seen in the lateral view. There is much too much right heart and too little left heart shadow in the PA view, indicating a swing of the lower part of the mediastinum to the right. The trachea is in its normal position. The right heart border is quite often still visible in the PA view in RML atelectasis because there is not enough airless lung lying against the heart to obscure it.

Patient **F** has densities on both sides of the heart, smudging its right and left borders and indicating lung density in both the RML and the lingula of the left upper lobe (LUL). There may also be some patchy involvement in the lower lobes, but it does not coalesce enough to obscure the diaphragm posteriorly.

Patient **I** has partial collapse of the left upper lobe that has obscured the left heart border and shifted the mediastinum sharply to the left. The whole left lung *could not* be atelectatic because the left leaf of the diaphragm is so clearly seen. This must mean the left *lower* lobe (LLL) is well aerated. This patient had an obstructing carcinoma of the LUL bronchus. There was also a mass of nodes at the left hilum, seen vaguely outlined here by air in the lower lobe.

Nobody has a right upper lobe (RUL) collapse.

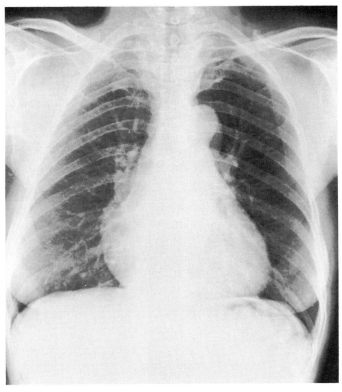

Figure 1–104

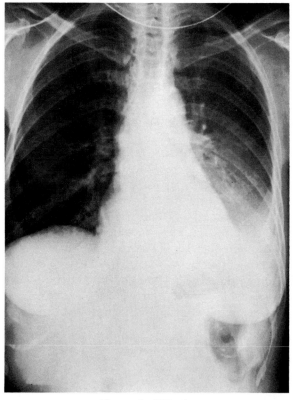

Figure 1-105   A

Problems

At the left you have two patients with fever whose PA chest films show left lower lung field densities of some kind. A systematic analysis of the PA films alone should inform you (1) what part of the lung is involved, and (2) how the related left laterals would differ from each other.

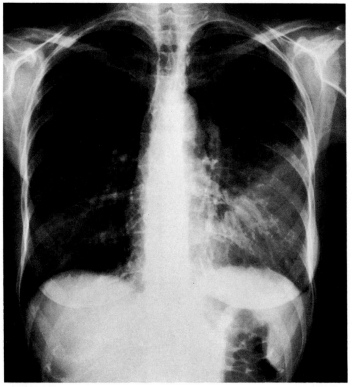

Figure 1-106   B

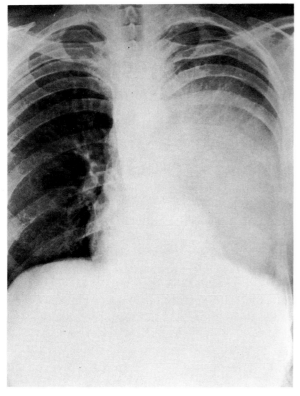

Figure 1–107 C

Problems

Here you have two more patients with trouble on the left side. Analyze their PA views with regard to degree of inspiration, rotation if any, mediastinal shift if any, and lobe involved. Predict the related left lateral chest films.

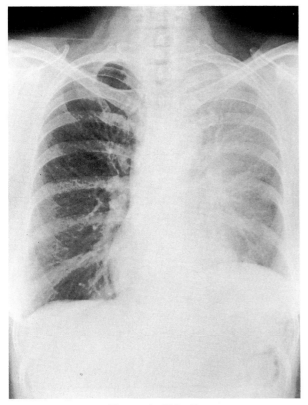

Figure 1–108 D

Answers to Page 50

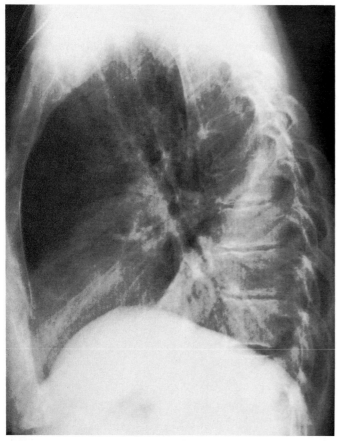

Figure 1–109   A

Mrs. **A** has a lower lung field density that obscures the diaphragm but not the heart border.

The dark shadow of the left lower lobe bronchus is *also* seen to extend downward across the heart border, suggesting that it may have consolidated lung tissue surrounding it (an air bronchogram). There are, therefore, three roentgen findings on this single film to suggest left *lower* lobe consolidation: lost diaphragmatic interface, heart/lung interface preserved, and an air bronchogram involving the lower lobe bronchus.

The left lateral film (Fig. 1–109) shows a wedge of density overlying the lower thoracic vertebrae bounded anteriorly by the slanting major fissure and only one visible diaphragm (the normal right). Note the air bronchogram, but do not be confused by the fact that you are *also* seeing white branching trunks; these represent the normal vascular supply to the *right* lower lobe surrounded by air!

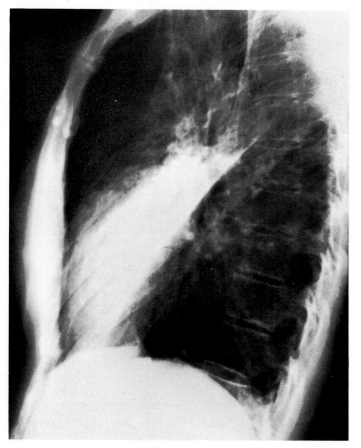

Figure 1–110   B

Mrs. **B** has a lung density that obscures the heart border but not the diaphragm, roentgen findings that should at once suggest to you consolidation of the anterior part of the lung lying against the heart (i.e., the lingular division of the left upper lobe). The related lateral film (Fig. 1–110) shows the anticipated white wedge overlying the heart shadow.

Be sure to study the two problem PA films matched against the two laterals by placing the margin of page 52 in the middle of page 51.

Answers to Page 51

(Now place the margin of page 51 in the center seam.)

Patient **C** has left lower lobe consolidation in spite of the presence of clear interface boundaries for both heart and diaphragm (Fig. 1–111). This may often be so when there is some atelectasis of the lower lobe so that the major fissure is displaced posteriorly and the lingula somewhat overexpanded. In Patient **A** the PA view was made leaning farther forward. In Patient **C** there is a marked degree of kyphosis present so that the lower lobe "lives" farther back in the chest. Remember then that the heart border is a more dependable index than the diaphragm in the PA view in questions of lower lobe involvement and that the disappearance of the posterior segment of left diaphragm in the lateral clinches the matter in patients like Mr. **C**. (He also has a hiatus hernia, by the way, with a fluid level above the diaphragm.)

Patient **D** has a very high left diaphragm, clearly seen, and her left heart border is obscured. This should immediately suggest collapse of the left upper lobe, and the lateral film (Fig. 1–112) confirms that interpretation of the findings (the crescentic wedge of density against the sternum overlying part of the heart shadow). Its sharp posterior border indicates the position of the major fissure and the anterior margin of the overexpanded left lower lobe. Note two diaphragmatic shadows and the normal spine density compared with Figure 1–111.

Patients **A, B,** and **C** had pneumonia clinically and recovered. Patient **D** had an obstructing carcinoma of the left upper lobe bronchus with mediastinal metastases involving the phrenic nerve and a paralyzed left diaphragm.

(Be sure to study the differences between the four laterals on pages 52 and 53 together.)

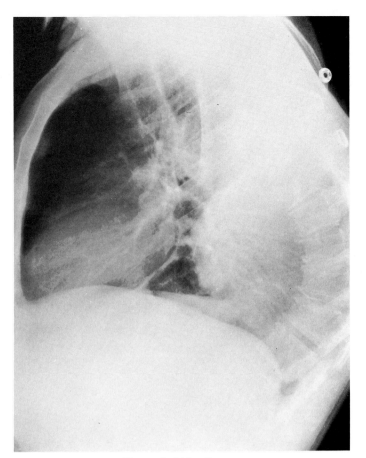

Figure 1–111 C

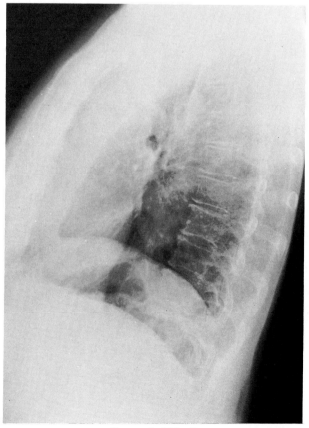

Figure 1–112 D

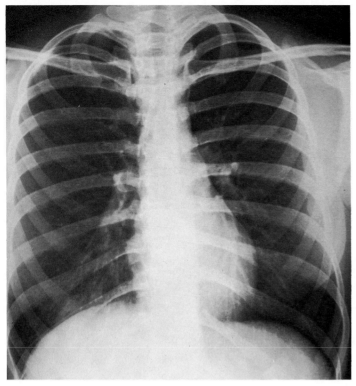

Figure 1-113 A

Problems

Five particularly desirable prospective technical employees for your hospital come up for review medically, and you have to decide whether they should be hired.

A, B, D, and **E** have positive skin tests with medium-strength PPD. **C** is negative but has some nontender cervical nodes and you think you can feel his spleen. He is coughing but afebrile. **A** and **E** have slight elevations of temperature and **E** also coughs, although he is obviously a chain smoker.

Here are their chest films. (The radiologist's reports have been withheld and you are on your own.) Examine their films, interspace for interspace, using any other films in the book as norm controls, and decide what you would recommend. Remember that good technicians are hard to find and each of these five people is badly wanted by one of your laboratories, no equally well-trained applicants being available.

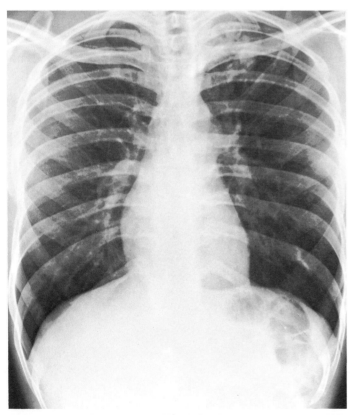

Figure 1-114   B

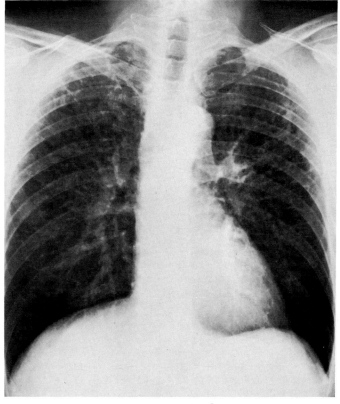

Figure 1-115   C

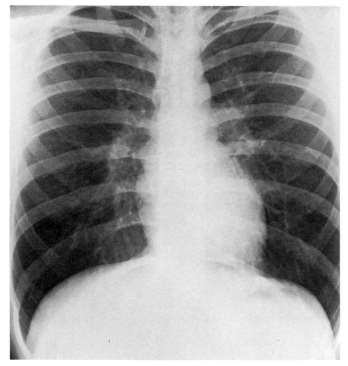

Figure 1-116   D

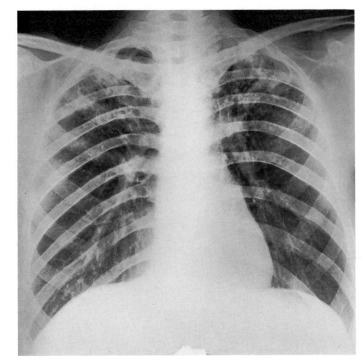

Figure 1-117   E

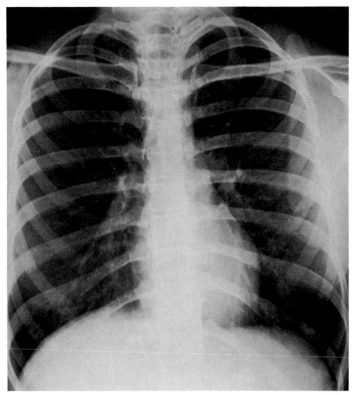

Figure 1–118   A

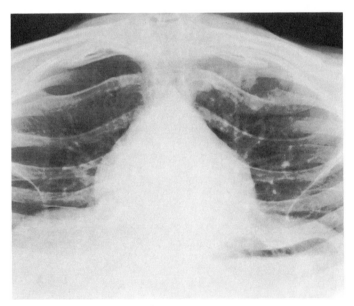

Figure 1–119   B

Answers

Applicant **A** has a patch of density in the ninth interspace close to the right diaphragm. There is nothing like it in the corresponding interspace on the left. The rest of this young woman's chest film is normal. On further questioning she said she had not been feeling very well for a week before the film was made. This is a very unlikely location for tuberculosis (not impossible—just very improbable). Figure 1–118 shows you her check film. In the interval of 12 days the patch has almost completely cleared. This patient was judged to have had a minor unrecognized bronchopneumonia clearing without treatment and was hired. She was followed carefully for a year in good health and did not develop obvious active tuberculosis.

Applicant **B** is another story. In the classic upper lobe location for tuberculosis this patient has a soft, cloudy density on the left. An apical lordotic film (Fig. 1–119) confirms its presence. Of course, bacteriologic confirmation is essential to a diagnosis. This patient should probably not be employed anywhere for a few weeks while the lesion is being treated.

Applicant **C,** with his nontender nodes, questionable spleen, negative skin test, and persistent cough without fever does not suggest tuberculosis clinically. His chest film shows a fine linear infiltration throughout both lung fields, rather diffuse and uniform in distribution. The hila are in normal position and seem rather thickened though not definitely nodular. Biopsy of a node confirmed the clinical suspicion of sarcoidosis. The patient was placed on therapy and employed. He made an excellent recovery and a chest film two years later appeared entirely normal.

Applicant **D** has a normal chest film. He was in excellent general health without symptoms of any kind. A positive PPD at age 20, however, is considered by many to indicate minimal active tuberculosis of undetermined site. Further questioning revealed recent exposure to tuberculosis, and he was treated prophylactically. The young man was hired with the proviso that he agree to treatment.

Applicant **E** has bilateral infiltrative densities also in the upper lobes. In addition there are round, white-margined radiolucent areas on both sides that suggest cavities. Note, too, that the vascular trunks to the lower lobes have an appearance suggesting that they are stretched, and the hila seem high in relation to the heart shadow. This generally implies a very considerable decrease in size of the upper lobes, retraction from scarring rather than atelectasis. The upper lobes are probably, therefore, much more involved than they appear to be on first inspection. Although tuberculosis is never actually a roentgen diagnosis but rather a bacteriologic one, here the radiologist will undoubtedly inform you (perhaps in the way he phrases his report) that there is a 99 per cent probability that you will find this patient has bilateral active upper lobe tuberculosis and a positive sputum. His employment should be delayed.

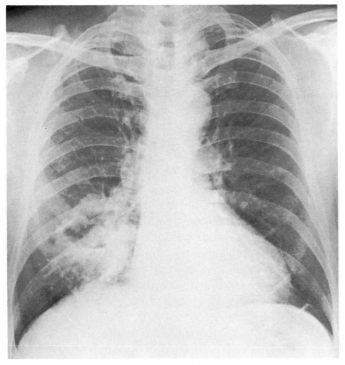

Figure 1–120 John C.

Problems

You have five patients with productive cough and bloody sputum. The three women are febrile; the men are not.

Study their films carefully and then check out the *roentgen findings* listed below, entering the initial of the patient's surname in the appropriate blank. If the finding is not present on any film, enter a zero.

_____ HAS A THIN-WALLED CAVITY AND A CALCIFIED PRIMARY COMPLEX.

_____ SHOWS A SIGNIFICANT DEGREE OF ROTATION.

_____ = THE NUMBER OF PATIENTS IN THIS GROUP WHOSE ACTIVE LESION MUST BE IN THE UPPER LOBE.

_____ HAS A STRAIGHT LINE THAT COULD BE EITHER A FLUID LEVEL WITHIN A LARGE LOWER LOBE CAVITY *OR* THE MINOR FISSURE WITH SOLID LUNG BENEATH IT IN THE MIDDLE LOBE.

_____ HAS MEDIASTINAL SHIFT.

_____ HAS A MASS DENSITY WHICH COULD NOT BE ENTIRELY IN THE RIGHT MIDDLE LOBE.

_____ = THE NUMBER OF CAVITIES IN FIGURE 1–124.

_____ HAS A THIN-WALLED CAVITY AND FLUID LEVEL BEHIND THE LEFT VENTRICLE AGAINST THE DIAPHRAGM.

_____ HAS A LUCENT AREA SUGGESTING A CAVITY IN THE LEFT UPPER LOBE.

_____ HAS A CAVITY WITH AN IRREGULAR WALL SUGGESTING BROKEN-DOWN TUMOR.

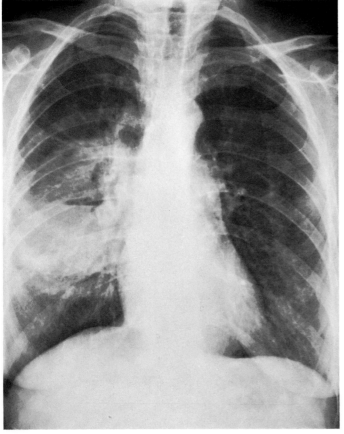

Figure 1–121 Amanda T.

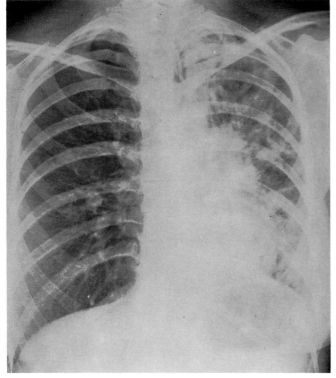

Figure 1–122   Mary A.

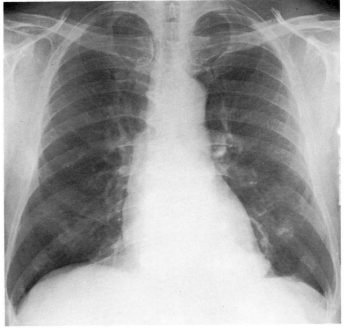

Figure 1–123   Richard V.

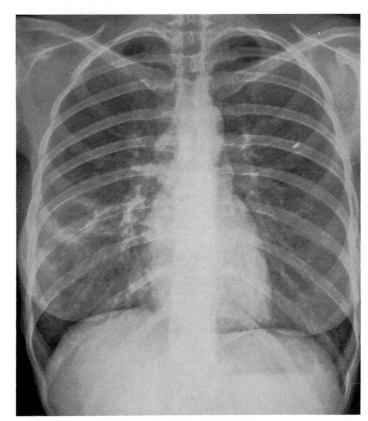

Figure 1–124   Adelaide N.

Answers

If you have made all the right decisions, you have a vertical acrostic that spells "cavitation" . . . upside down.

John C. is a man in his sixties, as suggested by the prominent uncoiled aorta and left ventricle. He was afebrile but coughing up a copious bloody sputum. His film shows a broken-down lesion, probably in the right lower lobe. The wall of the abscess is irregular in thickness and there are rounded masses projecting into the central cavity. At surgery a necrotic excavated carcinoma was found.

Amanda T., admitted with fever and bloody sputum, has some sort of straight-line interface extending out from her right hilum. This might be the minor fissure with consolidated right middle lobe below it. However, the density in her right lung extends upward too far to *limit* it to the middle lobe. There are two possible explanations: either she has two separate areas of consolidation (one in the middle lobe and one behind it in the apex of the lower lobe) *or* the straight line represents a fluid level in a large abscess in the apex of the lower lobe and the middle lobe is clear. The lateral film (Fig. 1–125) gives you the answer.

Richard V. has a normal chest film except for the fluid level behind the heart. Figure 1–126 is his lateral film. Any fluid- and air-filled structure near the midline and especially near the diaphragm brings the esophagus into question. A swallow of barium proved this to be a hiatus hernia. Mr. V.'s cough and sputum were later shown to relate to bronchiectasis, seldom visible on plain chest films like these.

Mary A., with fever and bloodstreaked sputum, clearly has left upper lobe involvement with a cavity in the fourth interspace just below the mid clavicle. The left upper lobe must be involved because the trachea is shifted to the left (there is no rotation). The sputum was positive for acid-fast bacilli and the patient never responded well to therapy. Figure 1–127 is her chest film a year later, with the left lower lobe now also involved. Figure 1–128 is a specimen radiograph of her inflated lungs at autopsy with the arterial supply injected with contrast material. Normal vessels are present on the right. There are no vessels in the left upper lobe. The vessels of the left lower lobe are diffusely abnormal. Extensive inflammatory changes may destroy the alveolar spaces and the pulmonary vasculature. Often in response to inflammatory changes, bronchial arterial hypertrophy occurs and supplies the abnormal lung.

Adelaide N. has a soft, thin-walled abscess cavity in her right lung and a calcified primary complex in her left, overlying the sixth rib. The location of the cavity (lower part of upper lobe or in lower lobe) is an unusual one for tuberculosis in a patient with clear upper lobes. From its roentgen appearance this could just as well be a nonspecific lung abscess, but the mediastinal shadow is slightly widened and the hila suggest nodular thickening. The sputum was found to be loaded with acid-fast bacilli.

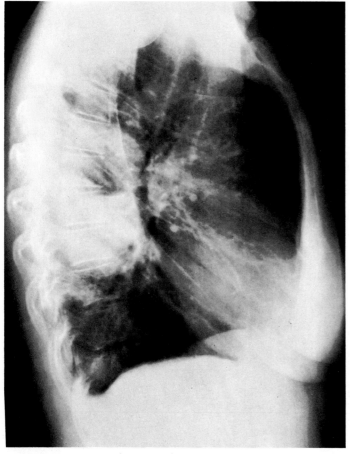

Figure 1–125 Amanda T.

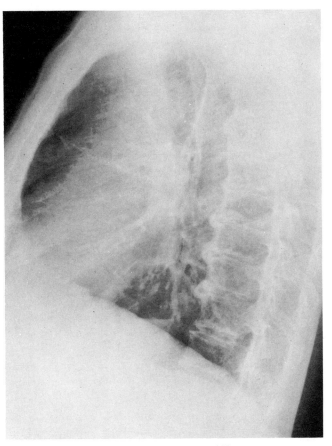

Figure 1–126   Richard V.

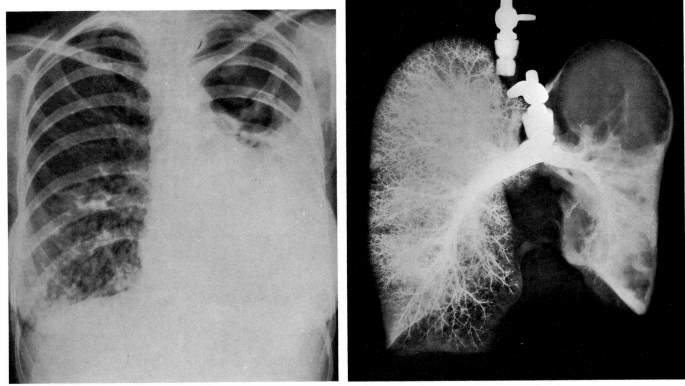

Figure 1–127   Mary A.

Figure 1–128

FOUR PATIENTS PRESENTING WITH CNS SYMPTOMS

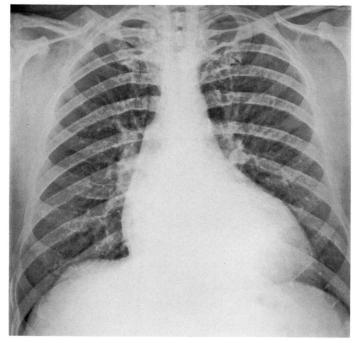

Figure 1–129 Mr. Alexander, age 35.

Mr. Alexander, an accountant, consults you because of fainting spells, sometimes preceded by dizziness. Twice in the past six months he has been found unconscious and convulsing at the top of the subway stairs on his way home from work. He had rheumatic fever at age 16 and knows he has had a murmur ever since.

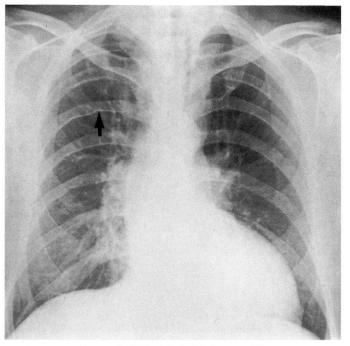

Figure 1–130 Mr. Baldwin, age 55.

Mr. Baldwin, a retired linotype operator, has had no medical attention of any kind for years and has no past medical history of interest. He comes to clinic now because of several episodes of pulsatile headache produced by exercise. The headache always disappears after rest, but he then develops numbness and a pins-and-needles sensation in his right hand and in the right side of his mouth. His mouth twitches and he sometimes has trouble finding words.

Mr. Perkins, a truckdriver, says he has been a heavy drinker since age 17. His fiancée will not marry him unless he stops drinking. Several times in the past three months he has stopped, and each time he has had several grand mal seizures within 24 hours, relieved when he began drinking again.

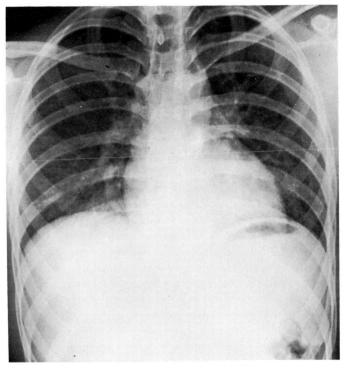

Figure 1–131 Mr. Perkins, age 25.

Mr. Bromson, a bookmaker, says he had an episode of profound dizziness with nausea and vomiting one month ago that gradually cleared over a period of several days during which everything "started spinning" whenever he turned his head to the right. A week ago on his way home from the track he fainted at the wheel of his car and had an automobile accident caused by his running into Mr. Perkins' truck, which was passing on his left.

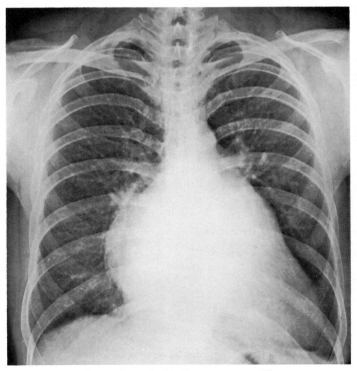

Figure 1–132 Mr. Bromson, age 35.

Answers

(Place margin of Page 64 in the middle of Page 62.)

AORTIC STENOSIS WITH STOKES-ADAMS SYNDROME

Mr. Alexander had a loud systolic murmur heard best in the second right interspace and transmitted into the neck. Neurologic examination was normal. A diagnosis of effort-initiated Stokes-Adams syncopal attacks was made because of insufficient perfusion of the brainstem and vestibular nuclei in periods of prolonged asystole. The film shows left ventricular preponderance, a small aorta, and engorged hila. Even in the absence of rib-notching, the whole picture might have been consistent with coarctation of the aorta rather than aortic stenosis, except that blood pressures were entirely within normal limits and uniform, with good femoral pulses. The auscultatory findings and his history of rheumatic fever make clear a diagnosis of pure rheumatic aortic stenosis with ventricular hypertrophy and Stokes-Adams episodes.

HIGH COARCTATION OF THE AORTA; ISCHEMIA OF LEFT CEREBRUM

Mr. Baldwin had a blood pressure (BP) of 170/100 in the right arm but much lower pressures in the left arm and both legs. Femoral pulses were very faint but present, presumably because of the very extensive collateral circulation, which was evident with pulsating vessels around the right scapula. The coarctation must be high and involve the ostium of the left carotid in view of the findings and the story, which implies ischemia of the left parietal and frontal lobes (tingling and expressive aphasia). Note the notching of ribs predominantly on the right. The patient died a month later at home of cerebral hemorrhage.

(Now place the margin of page 63 in the center seam between pages 64 and 65.)

NORMAL CHEST FILM AT EXPIRATION; "RUM FITS"

Mr. Perkins has been having seizures in response to withdrawal of alcohol. Except for a poor inspiration, his chest film is normal. (Figure 1–133 is his inspiration film.)

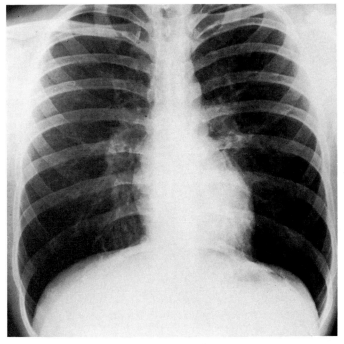

Figure 1–133

RHEUMATIC HEART DISEASE WITH EMBOLI TO THE BRAIN

Mr. Bromson obviously has advanced rheumatic heart disease with a greatly dilated left atrium and hypertrophied left ventricle. His first heart sound was replaced by a loud blowing systolic murmur with no opening snap, and he was fibrillating. At postmortem he was found to have multiple cerebral emboli.

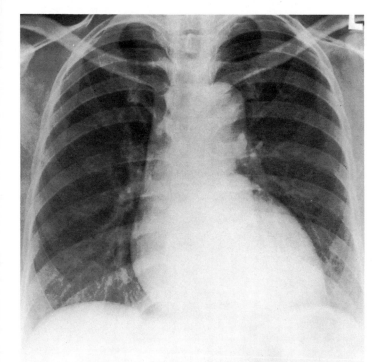

Figure 1–134   Mrs. Babcock, age 43.

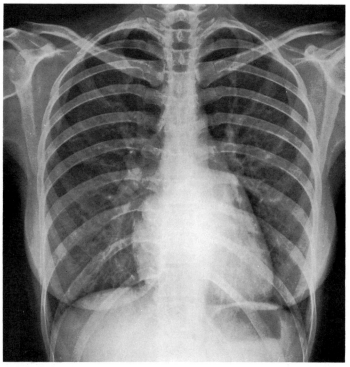

Figure 1–135   Mrs. Clayton, age 24.

FOUR PATIENTS ADMITTED TO MEDICINE FROM THE CLINIC

Are the following *roentgen findings* present on any of these films?

One-liter pleural effusion.
Prominent aortic knob.
Widened aorta, both ascending and descending.
Calcification which could be pericardial.
Engorged hilar vessels and increased vascular markings.
Pronounced cardiac enlargement.
Rotation off the sagittal plane.
Valid mediastinal shift.
Dilated superior vena cava.
Convex left cardiac border.
Missing rib.

The *historical items* below *might* be appropriate to which?

Sudden chest pain and dyspnea, three hours.
Pulsatile headaches three months.
Heart murmur since childhood.
Back pain and hematuria.
Abdominal swelling without ankle edema.
Rheumatic fever at age ten.

The following *physical signs* could fit which?

BP 230/110 both arms and even higher in both legs.

Markedly increased venous pressure of 35.

Presystolic murmur.

Quiet heart with decreased amplitude of pulsations at fluoroscopy.

Fibrillation.

Hepatomegaly.

Ankle edema.

Dyspnea on exertion.

Dyspnea at rest.

Electrocardiogram (ECG) shows low-voltage QRS complexes.

ECG normal.

ECG shows notched P waves.

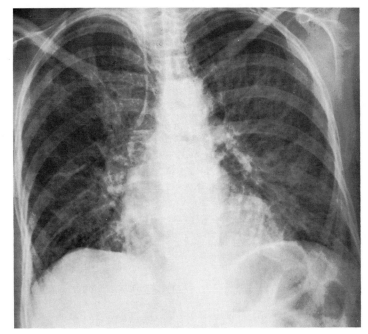

Figure 1–136   Mr. Archer, age 51.

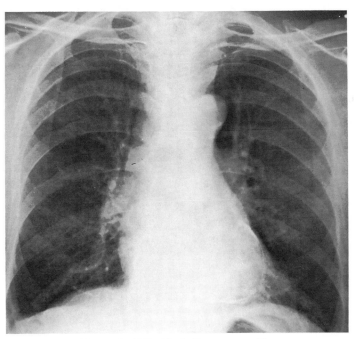

Figure 1–137   Mr. Belknap, age 65.

Answers

RENAL HYPERTENSION

Mrs. Babcock had hypertension of 230/110, and very severe headaches that had developed within a period of three months. She also complained of right back pain and had some microscopic hematuria. The selective renal angiogram (Fig. 1–138) showed an aneurysm of the right renal artery that was revised surgically with remission of the hypertension. The selective right renal arteriogram was done because of elevated renin value found in the right renal vein when it was catheterized. Her chest film shows cardiac enlargement with a prominent left ventricle and a generally widened aorta. She was not in failure.

RHEUMATIC HEART DISEASE

Mrs. Clayton had had rheumatic fever in childhood and had always known she had a murmur. She, too, had back pain and hematuria and was thought to have cast a renal embolus. She was fibrillating and had classic murmurs for mitral stenosis (MS) and mitral insufficiency (MI). Her film shows, besides the convex left heart border, an elevated left main bronchus and the dense shadow of the left atrium seen through the heart and projecting to the right.

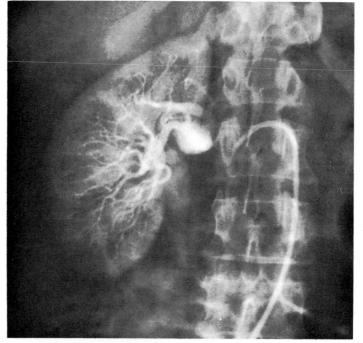

Figure 1–138 Mrs. Babcock.

MYOCARDIAL INFARCTION IN ACUTE CONGESTIVE FAILURE

Mr. Archer has engorged hilar and pulmonary vessels. He presented about four hours after onset of acute chest pain and was dyspneic at rest. The ECG was normal at the time this film was made, but by the time the heart failure had responded to therapy and Figure 1–139 was made the ECG indicated a recent myocardial infarction. His liver was never enlarged and he had no ascites. His film is rotated off the sagittal plane and the aorta is slightly uncoiled; hence, the suggestion of mediastinal shift must be discounted.

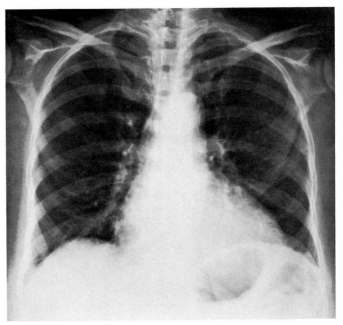

Figure 1–139 Mr. Archer.

CONSTRICTIVE PERICARDITIS

Mr. Belknap has calcification about the heart in two projections, implying that it must be diffusely distributed in a shell encasing the ventricles. (Figure 1–140 is his lateral; there are traces of barium in the esophagus not to be mistaken for part of the calcification.) He presented with ascites without ankle edema, hepatomegaly, dyspnea on exertion only, and distended neck veins. His superior vena cava appears distended on the chest film and his systemic venous pressure was elevated. A diagnosis of constrictive pericarditis was confirmed by echocardiography. (Although calcification of the pericardium does not necessarily imply constriction, the syndrome of constriction *is* very common in patients with large amounts of calcium.)

Nobody has a missing rib or pleural effusion.

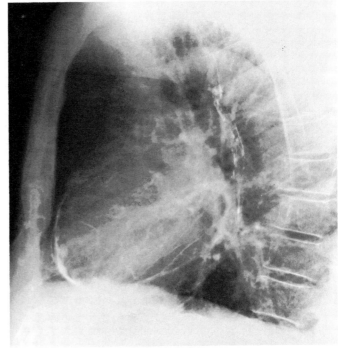

Figure 1–140 Mr. Belknap.

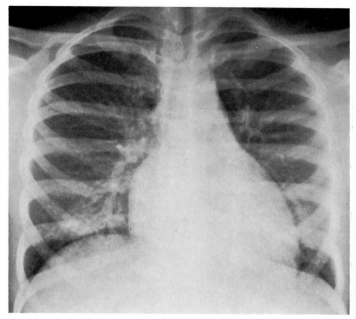

Figure 1–141   Mr. Duane.

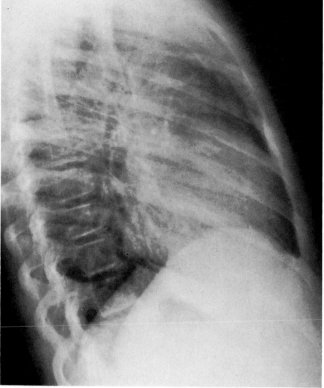

Figure 1–142   Mr. Duane.

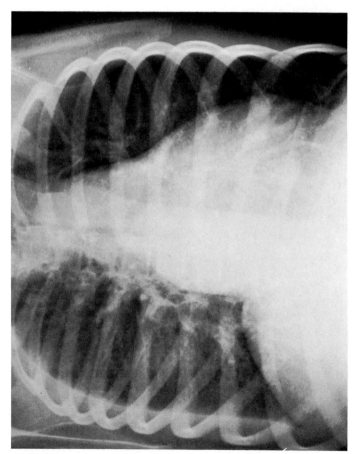

Figure 1–143   Mr. Duane.

Reconciling Conflicting Roentgen Evidence

In this exercise you have two patients whose various films have to be reconciled with each other *because roentgen evidence is conflicting.*

Which pieces of evidence are most convincing and how can you explain others that do not seem to agree with them?

Figure 1–143 must be interpreted at variance with Figures 1–141 and 1–142—why?

Figure 1–145 belies the pathology at first suggested by Figure 1–144—why?

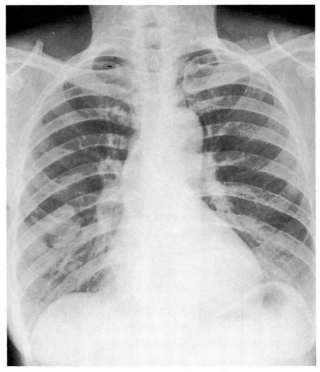

Figure 1–144 Mrs. Abernathy.

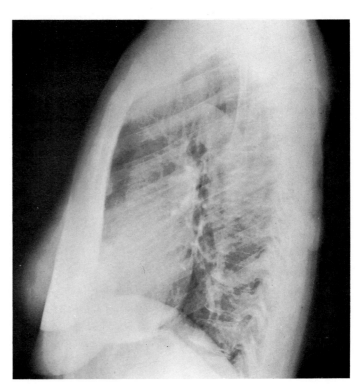

Figure 1–145 Mrs. Abernathy.

Answers

Mr. Duane's diaphragms are at the eighth rib on his PA film and you may have been tempted to discount his cardiac enlargement for that reason. Perhaps you noted that in the lateral film the top of the stomach bubble is quite distant from the dome of the left diaphragm; something must be occupying that space! There is no fluid whatever in the two sharp posterior angles on the lateral nor in the costophrenic sinuses in the PA view. However, the decubitus film *definitely* shows fluid separating lung from chest wall, indicating without any possible question the presence of pleural fluid. After a check to make certain all three films were made on the same patient (they were) you must conclude that the right diaphragmatic shadows in the PA and lateral films are actually fluid imprisoned underneath the lung and above the diaphragm. The patient was going into heart failure and had had several other attacks of cardiac insufficiency.

Mrs. Abernathy shows several sharply margined nodules in the right lung field below the level of the hilum. Examination of the lung area on the lateral film fails to reveal anything to correspond with their size, shape, and location. After checking the unit numbers to make sure this is indeed her lateral chest film, you restudy the film more closely and note the knobby appearance of the soft tissues of the back. Examination of the patient herself reveals three superficial neurofibromas below the right scapula.

In studying radiographs you must realize that *all* the roentgen findings have to be reconciled to your satisfaction. Apparent inconsistencies may sometimes be explained as technical, may sometimes result in the unscrambling of mislabeled films, and at other times may lead to a closer study of the films at hand and a diagnostic possibility not previously entertained.

Special Exercise (No Films)

What would be your conclusion if each of the following patients had had a single, perfectly normal PA chest film made at deep inspiration yesterday?

1. A man of 50 with an ECG showing evidence of a recent posterior myocardial infarction of some importance.

2. A woman of 25 with bright red hemoptysis twice in the past week and a dry cough.

3. A man who has coughed for years without fever or loss of weight and raises a half cup of sputum every morning.

4. A man with periodic chest pain that radiates down his left arm.

5. A child who has coughed and wheezed since yesterday when he choked on some popcorn.

6. A man of 60 who coughs, has lost 15 pounds in weight, and says he has had pneumonia twice in the past three months.

Answers

A knowledge of the limitations of the roentgen method of investigation of disease is as important as an acquaintance with its helpful positive findings.

1. A myocardial infarction may not give rise to any change in the efficiency of the heart function, and the chest film could remain normal throughout the episode.

2. Bright red hemoptysis and cough may indicate early active tuberculosis that is still invisible on the PA chest film. It may also go with a bronchial adenoma in a young woman, or, of course, any other cause of bleeding in the upper respiratory tract.

3. The history suggests bronchiectasis, which is usually hard to visualize on plain films of the chest without computed tomography.

4. Coronary insufficiency and anginal pain may be associated with a normal cardiac configuration on the chest film.

5. Nonopaque foreign bodies may act as check valves, obstructing the egress but not the ingress of air through one main bronchus. There is frequently a stage at which the mediastinum is in the midline at full inspiration though it deviates far to the uninvolved side with each expiration. Hence, a single film made at inspiration may be entirely normal. You should request an expiration film.

6. Bronchogenic carcinoma may cause repeated episodes of atelectasis, sometimes mistaken for pneumonia.

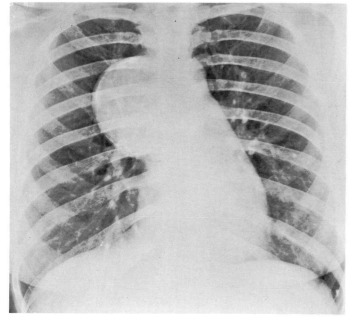

Figure 1–146 Mrs. Davidson, age 32.

FOUR PATIENTS WITH MEDIASTINAL MASSES

Mrs. Davidson consults you because of a cough without fever for three weeks, headaches brought on by smelling bacon cooking, an aching pain in her left knee at night, and attacks of nausea and vomiting whenever her husband calls her from his mother's apartment where he goes once a week for dinner. On being asked whether her cough yields any sputum, she insists that from time to time she has coughed up red hair. She has red hair, blue eyes, and very white skin.

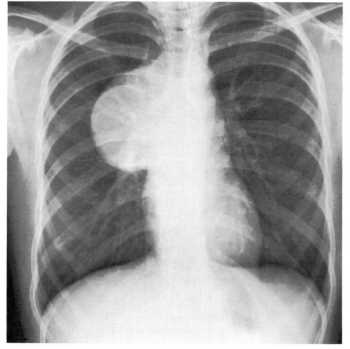

Figure 1–147 Nancy Porter, age 10.

Nancy Porter is brought in by her parents who are worried because she wakes up at night crying and complaining of back pain. This usually happens after an active day and has been going on for about two years, but a careful check-up (which did not include a chest film, however) had been entirely negative a year ago at the Army Base where Sgt. Porter was stationed.

Mr. Rankin, too, consults you because of back pain, more or less constant, throbbing in character, and localized to the midthoracic spine.

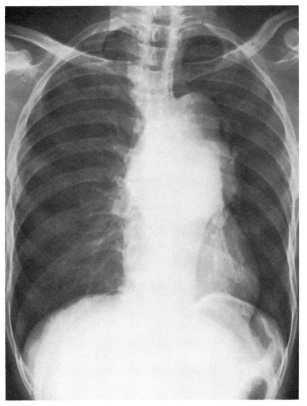

Figure 1–148 Mr. Rankin, age 50.

Miss Patterson has no complaints but has asked for a general physical exam prior to taking on several years of graduate study during which she will have to work days and go to school nights.

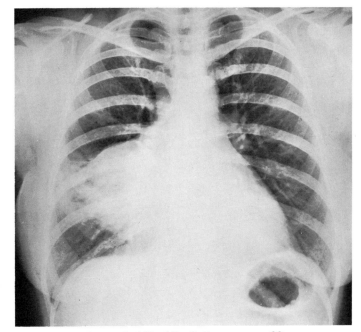

Figure 1–149 Miss Patterson, age 29.

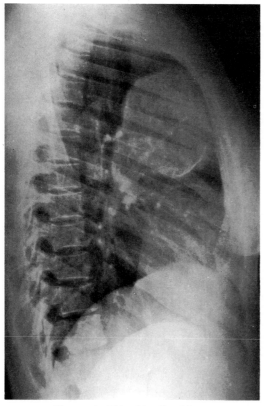

Figure 1–150   Mrs. Davidson.

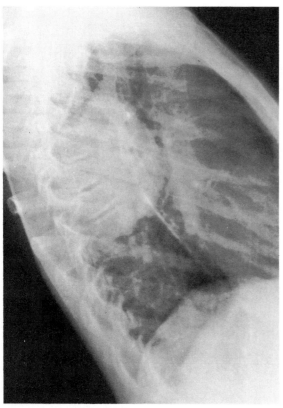

Figure 1–151   Nancy Porter.

Answers

Mrs. Davidson's left lateral film is Figure 1–150. She has a mediastinal mass that must be anterior because it clearly ablates the border of heart and aorta. This proved to be a dermoid cyst that communicated with the bronchus. It contained red hair, all of which goes to show that you should listen to the patient; he or she is telling you what is wrong and there *may* be one significant bit of information in the middle of an improbable tale.

Nancy Porter has a mediastinal mass, but the border of the ascending aorta may be seen through the mass. The hilar vessels can be seen superimposed on it, which always tells you the mass in not *in* the hilum but in front of or behind it. There is another finding of great importance: the medial portion of the posterior sixth rib is missing, suggesting bone erosion, which should also, of course, place the tumor far posterior in the chest. Note that the lateral (Fig. 1–151) confirms this, and that an AP Bucky detail (Fig. 1–152) shows erosion of ribs and vertebral bodies. Posterior mediastinal masses are most commonly neural in origin, and in young girls very frequently ganglioneuromas, the final operative diagnosis in Nancy.

Mr. Rankin has a posterior mediastinal mass, too, which seems to produce not only a bulge in the descending aorta (follow its lateral margin upward from the diaphragm) and widening of the aortic knob, but also a dense white shadow seen through the heart. In the lateral (Fig. 1–153) this again seems to be a part of the aorta and clearly erodes the anterior margins of two thoracic vertebrae. Figure 1–154, his angiogram, proves that the mass is vascular and an aortic aneurysm.

Miss Patterson had a pericardial cyst (Fig. 1–155); this was proved at surgery.

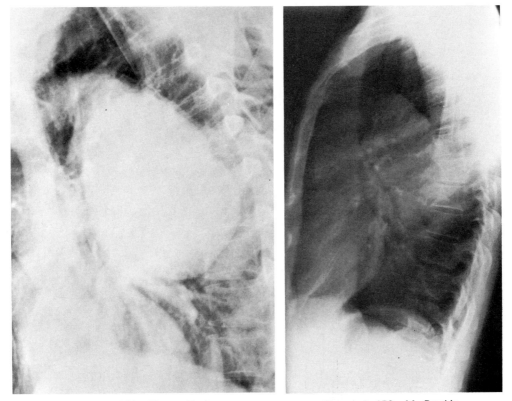

Figure 1–152   Nancy Porter.   Figure 1–153   Mr. Rankin.

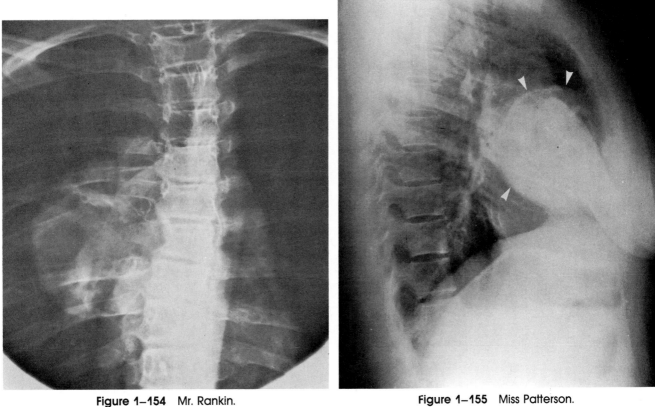

Figure 1–154   Mr. Rankin.   Figure 1–155   Miss Patterson.

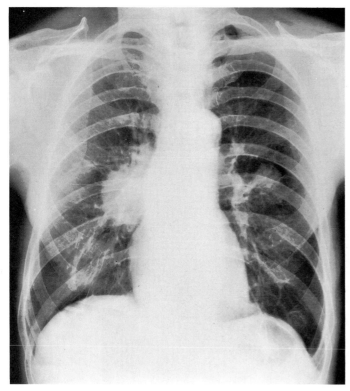

Figure 1-156   Mr. Astor.

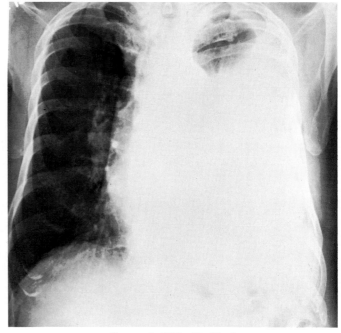

Figure 1-157   Mr. Nash.

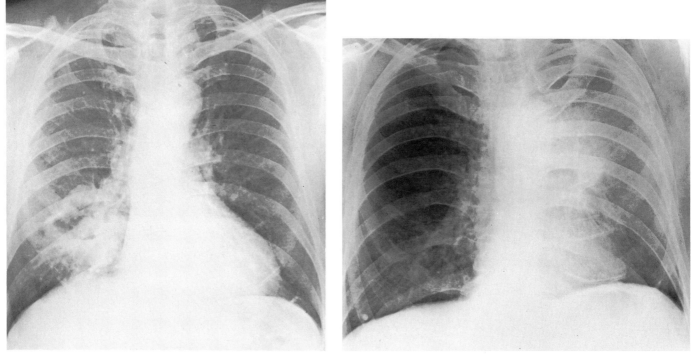

Figure 1-158   Mr. Ireland.

Figure 1-159   Mr. Casper.

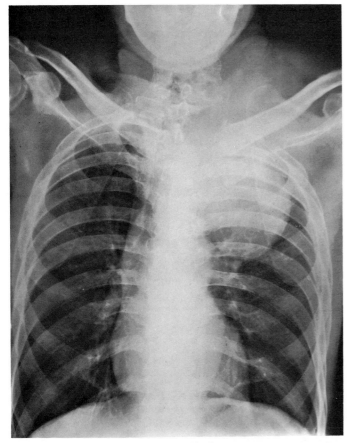

Figure 1–160 Mr. Rogers.

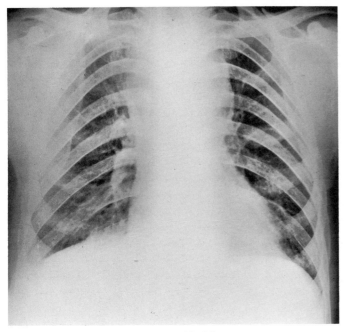

Figure 1–161 Mr. Mayer.

SIX MEN WITH CHEST SYMPTOMS

FOLLOW DIRECTIONS PRECISELY

1. First study the films carefully and note all *roentgen findings* you can be certain of before reading any farther.
2. Then try to decide what symptoms each man reported to his doctor.
3. Then tally the particular nine roentgen findings listed below with the initial of the appropriate patient's last name (zero if none fits).
4. Finally, decide what disease entity *could* have been the final pathologic diagnosis in all six men.

Specific Roentgen Findings

_____ EROSION RIGHT POSTERIOR SEVENTH RIB.

_____ MEDIASTINAL SHIFT TO THE LEFT.

_____ EROSION OF RIBS AND VERTEBRAE.

_____ THICK-WALLED ABSCESS SUGGESTING BROKEN-DOWN TUMOR.

_____ BILATERAL SUPERIOR MEDIASTINAL WIDENING.

_____ EVIDENCE OF COLLAPSE OF AN ENTIRE LUNG.

_____ HYDROTHORAX WITHOUT PNEUMOTHORAX.

_____ EVIDENCE FOR LEFT UPPER LOBE COLLAPSE.

_____ DISSEMINATED PULMONARY MASSES.

Answers

You should have a nice sense of satisfaction on completing the foregoing exercise. We hope that it has proved to you how much radiology you have learned. The tallying of a few of the specific roentgen findings present on these six chest films will have provided you with the word *acrimonca*, a vertical *(scrambled)* acrostic of *carcinoma*, the final diagnosis in all six patients.

Lung cancer has so wide a spectrum of roentgen findings and so varied a pattern of presenting complaints that it affords teachers of radiology a superb opportunity for review, not only of radiology but also of the pathophysiology of the disease.

All six patients had cough of some duration and weight loss. Only *Mr. Ireland's* cough was productive of much sputum, although both *Mr. Rogers* and *Mr. Casper* had had hemoptysis several times.

Mr. Astor and *Mr. Rogers* presented with back pain. *Mr. Astor's* pain was below the right scapula, sometimes radiating around to the front, and he was at first believed to have herpes zoster.

Mr. Rogers' pain was classic for lung cancer when it occurs close to the apex of the upper lobe (often called a Pancoast or superior sulcus tumor) and involves the brachial plexus. His pain was in the left shoulder and arm and he himself was concerned he might have angina. His film shows erosion of the posterior segments of the first three ribs and also of the left transverse processes and laminae of the first three thoracic vertebrae. (See Figure 1–162, a Bucky detail of the thoracic inlet.)

Mr. Nash and *Mr. Casper* presented with dyspnea, and *Mr. Mayer* said he "could not get his breath." He had stridor audible across the room and the distended neck veins seen with superior mediastinal syndrome. On examination he had a Horner's syndrome. His trachea and sympathetic chain were encircled by a mass of metastatic nodes. His primary

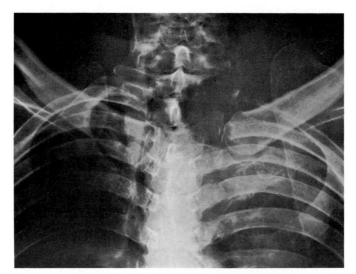

Figure 1–162 Bucky detail, Mr. Rogers.

tumor is not visible but was in the right upper lobe bronchus. (Faced with this kind of mediastinal widening or symptoms suggestive of a Pancoast tumor, the workup of suspected Pancoast tumor is best accomplished with magnetic resonance imaging [MRI] because MRI can precisely define tumor involving the superior sulcus with the nerve and vascular anatomy. Percutaneous biopsy usually can be used to diagnose cell type, followed by chemotherapy and radiation therapy. Surgical resection may subsequently be done.)

Mr. Nash had pleural seeding from the left lower lobe tumor you cannot see in the presence of so much pleural fluid. There were malignant cells in fluid taken during a diagnostic thoracentesis.

Mr. Casper had a carcinoma obstructing his left upper lobe bronchus and collapse of the lobe distal to the tumor as the imprisoned air was resorbed. There is little rotation, certainly not enough to explain the shift of both trachea and heart to the left. That none of the left heart border is seen implies airless left upper lobe lying against it. The well-visualized left diaphragm, on the other hand, tells you that the left lower lobe is inflated. (None of the six patients has roentgen evidence of collapse of a whole lung, of course.)

Mr. Astor has, in addition to his missing rib, a mass on the right and a smaller round mass in the left lung. His rib involvement is a lytic metastasis to bone rather than the erosion by contiguous extension of tumor you see in *Mr. Rogers*. The mass on the right was a primary bronchogenic carcinoma in the superior segment of the right lower lobe. (Note visible hilar vessels superimposed on it.) The mass in the left lung was a metastasis.

Of these six patients, only *Mr. Ireland* survived. His right lung and abscessed tumor were resected, and he was alive five years later without evidence of recurrence. Lung cancer is the most common form of cancer in women also.

Final Exercise on the Analysis of the Lateral Chest Film

No names, no ages, no presenting symptoms, no clinical story, not even the related PA views! Just the laterals to compare and analyze. There are ten of them on this page spread and the next. Jot down your findings on a piece of paper before you look at the answers, since to commit yourself to paper is enormously more instructive than a cursory verbal commitment.

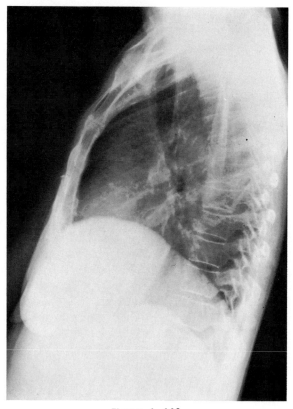

Figure 1–163

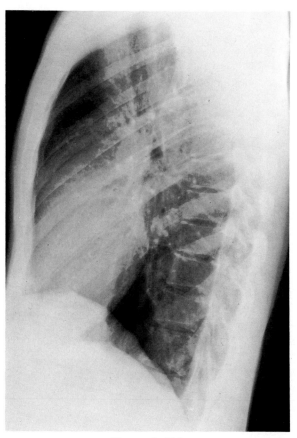

Figure 1–164

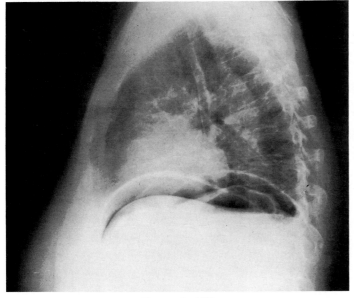

Figure 1–165

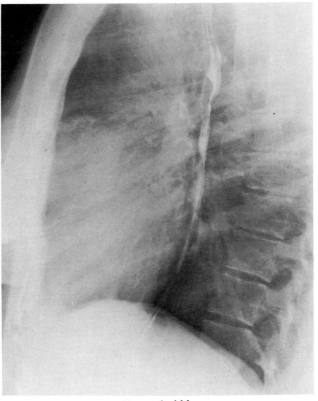

Figure 1–166

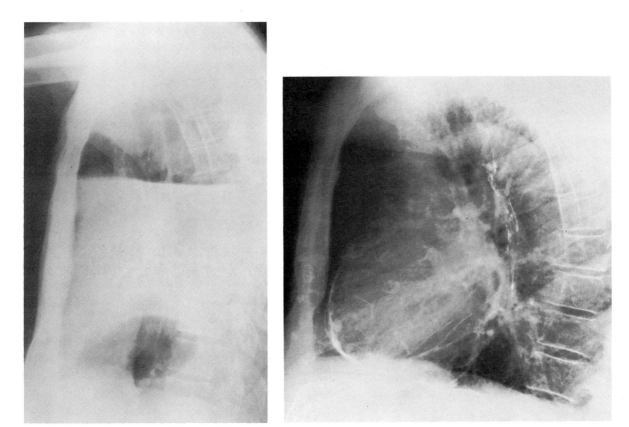

Figure 1–167

Figure 1–168

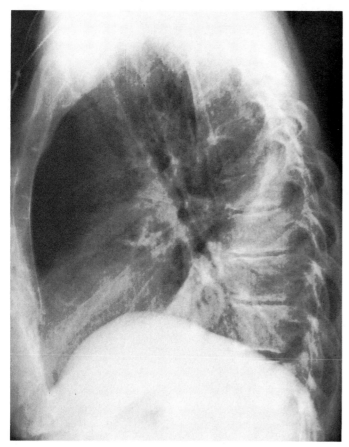

Figure 1-169

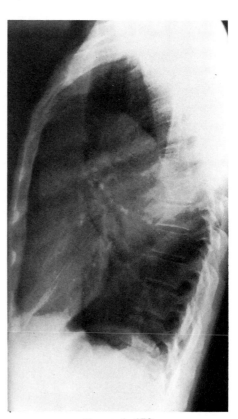

Figure 1-170

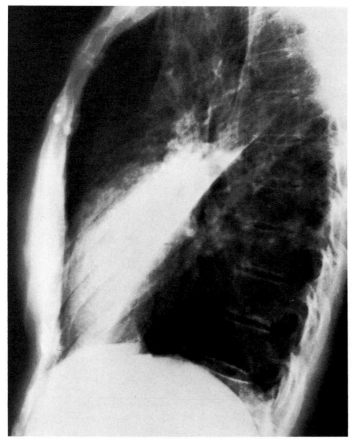

Figure 1-171

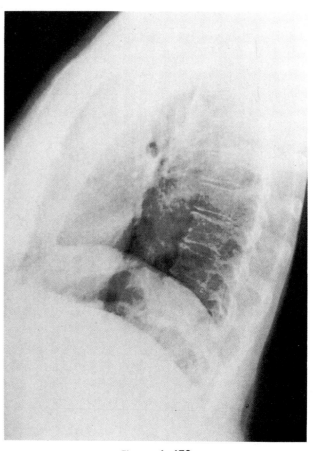

Figure 1-172

Answers

Fig. 1–163: High right diaphragm, big liver with metastases from colon carcinoma (repeat of Fig. 1–19).

Fig. 1–164: Normal left lateral (repeat of Fig. 1–18).

Fig. 1–165: Free peritoneal air under both diaphragms (repeat of Fig. 1–26).

Fig. 1–166: Thymoma in the anterior mediastinum (repeat of Fig. 1–30).

Fig. 1–167: Left hydropneumothorax (repeat of Fig. 1–46).

Fig. 1–168: Pericardial calcification (repeat of Fig. 1–140).

Fig. 1–169: Left lower lobe pneumonia (repeat of Fig. 1–109).

Fig. 1–170: Aortic aneurysm (repeat of Fig. 1–153).

Fig. 1–171: Left upper lobe pneumonia, lingular division (repeat of Fig. 1–110).

Fig. 1–172: Left upper lobe collapse (repeat of Fig. 1–112).

(Note: Both students and teachers should realize that because the eye tends to recognize any given film when it is studied a second time, the student has been at an advantage in this exercise. However, with a large number of films the advantage is principally one of increased confidence, on the whole a good thing. Now try some laterals cold!)

2 | Abdomen

Suggested Systematic Procedure for Examining Each Radiograph (Don't Just Gaze! Analyze!)

1. A properly exposed plain film of the abdomen will show in detail the anatomy of the lumbar vertebrae and will "burn out" the flanks, where there is less patient! Compare the overall density of the central third of the abdomen with the lateral thirds and bones. Is this, therefore, a well-penetrated or a poorly penetrated plain film? Is there any obvious reason why it should be overpenetrated (free peritoneal air? large amount of gas in intestine? thin patient?) or underpenetrated (ascites? obesity? fluid-filled loops of intestine? soft tissue masses?)?

2. Check the flank stripes and psoas margins for symmetry and normal sharp interfaces. The illustrations in this part of the book have been specially prepared so that you can see details in the flanks without "bright-lighting" them as you would have to do with an actual film.

3. Look for the splenic tip, the liver edge, and renal outlines. Are visible organ masses normal in size?

4. Identify: urinary bladder, perivesical fat, and rectal bubble.

5. Inspect the bones: pelvis, lumbar spine, ribs, and upper femora.

6. Identify all the air contained in bowel, noting stomach, small bowel, and large bowel collections which look different because of their variations in mucosal markings and structure. Is there too much air? too little? Are the collections of air displaced in any way?

7. Is there any "uncontained air"? (outside bowel? under the liver or lateral to it? in the bile ducts? under the diaphragm? in abscesses?)

8. Are there any calcifications, normal or anticipated for the patient's age, abnormal or unusual? rib cartilages; vessels; soft tissues; concretions in gallbladder or kidney; along course of ureters; over bladder, pancreas, or in the mesentery?

9. Don't forget to look at the bases of the lungs if they are included.

10. *Now*—are there any roentgen images or interfaces you cannot identify or define?

Note. A proper film study includes all of the above before you consider the clinical data, and then a reappraisal in view of the patient's presenting problem.

Note Also. Some of the illustrations in this volume will seem to you underpenetrated for technical reasons rather than for pathologic reasons. We and the publisher have arranged this intentionally so that all the more subtle contrast values would be present on the print, which, unlike the original film, cannot be transilluminated with a bright light.

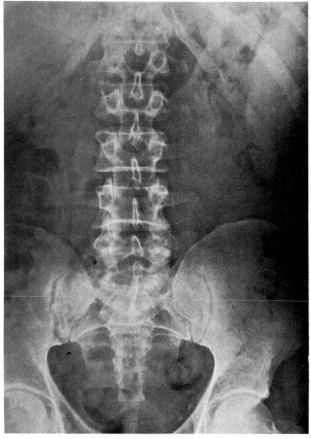

Figure 2–1 Mark Thyme

Mark Thyme, 28, electrician, comes to the hospital because he has been "doubled up" with waves of colic since yesterday afternoon. He has vomited twice, hates hospitals and all doctors, and insists it is "something I ate." Pain is midabdominal, not referred, and seems to be abating. You find normal bowel sounds and no localized tenderness or guarding. Rectal negative; temperature (T) 100.9° F; white blood count (WBC) 26,000.

Note: *All names, of course, are fictitious.*

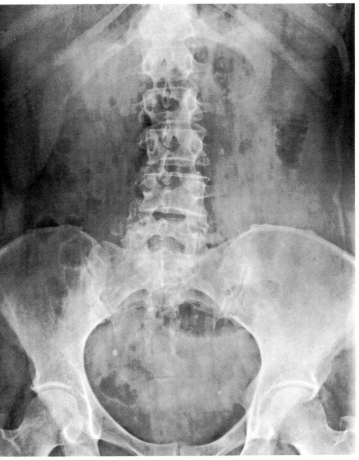

Figure 2–2　Magnolia Winter

Magnolia Winter, 43, homemaker, has also had severe abdominal cramps in her back and right side for 36 hours. She has vomited several times. The cramps have come in waves, lasting half an hour, with relief between. You find some tenderness high in the right upper quadrant (RUQ) but no guarding or masses. Peristalsis is normal and there is slight tenderness on the right by rectal. T 98.1° F; WBC 8500.

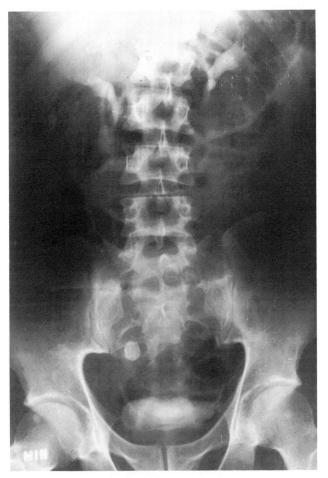

Figure 2–3　Phillip Penuche

Phillip Penuche, 33, automotive mechanic, has had moderately severe crampy midabdominal pain off and on for three days. It is now more localized to the right side and he vomited four times this morning. You find diffuse tenderness and some guarding in the right lower quadrant (RLQ) and there is a vague impression of an ill-defined mass. Rectal negative; T 98.6° F; WBC 18,000.

Answers

Mr. Thyme's diagnosis after another few hours seemed obviously that of an acute gastrointestinal upset from which he recovered promptly. The plain film shows no abnormality except definite splenomegaly, the stomach bubble being displaced to the right by the enlarged spleen. Complete hemogram showed acute myelogenous leukemia. (You missed the spleen on physical exam but spotted it on the radiograph and went back to feel again, especially in view of the white count.)

Mrs. Winter has no evidence of distended bowel loops. The tip of the spleen and liver border are seen and do not appear unusual; there is a small calcific density to the right of the sacrum that could be a low ureteral calculus. An excretory urogram at 30 minutes (Fig. 2–4) shows acute ureteral obstruction and an intense nephrogram with distended calices and ureter on the right. The stone was passed spontaneously the next day. The small calcific shadow near the left ischial spine is a phlebolith.

Mr. Penuche's story and elevated white blood cell count make imperative a consideration of appendicitis, and the physical findings suggest perforation and an appendiceal abscess. He also mentioned that he had noticed blood in his urine for a couple of days. He had an intravenous urogram (see Fig. 2–3), which shows a dense round calcification overlying the right sacrum. This is a large very prominent appendicolith. His urinary system was normal. The presence of an appendicolith in a symptomatic patient is indicative of acute appendicitis. Occasionally, urinary symptoms and even findings such as hematuria may accompany acute appendicitis. At surgery a gangrenous appendix was found with perforation and a periappendiceal abscess. The large appendicolith was found in the abscess.

Why people develop appendicitis is usually not known. Occasionally some ingested object may cause it as in a young boy who swallowed a straight pin while helping his mother (Fig. 2–5). He developed abdominal pain several weeks later. The supine abdominal film shows the metallic object: a straight pin. Figure 2–6 is a film from his barium enema that shows the pin lodged in the appendix. The oval surrounding soft tissue mass was found to be a foreign body granuloma at appendectomy. No perforation was found.

Note: *Throughout the book the layout allows you to tip and fold pages in order to view two films on the same patient together.*

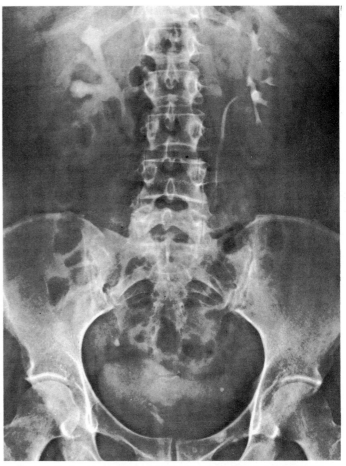

Figure 2–4   Mrs. Winter, 30-minute intravenous pyelogram.

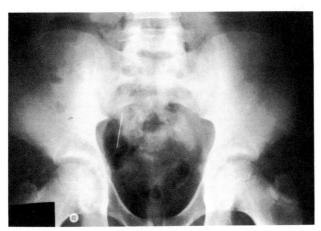

Figure 2–5   Appendicitis in a boy who swallowed a pin.

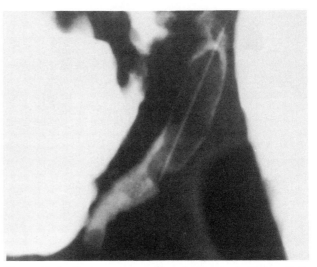

Figure 2–6   Barium enema film of the boy in Figure 2–5.

THREE PATIENTS WITH ABDOMINAL PAIN AND DISTENSION

Abraham Mixter, 54, sports reporter, has had crampy abdominal pain for 18 hours. His abdomen is distended, tympanitic, and tender but not rigid. You find increased peristalsis. Rectal negative; T 98.1° F; WBC 9000.

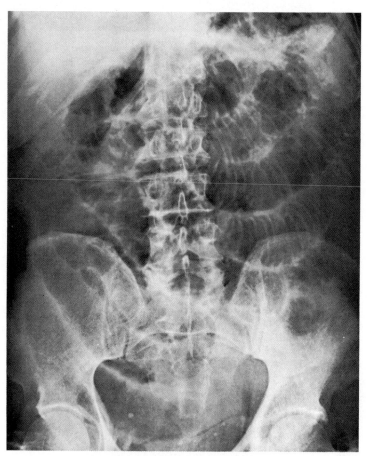

Figure 2–7   Abraham Mixter

Patrick Mahoney, 66, retired assemblyman, comes to medical clinic complaining of distension, crampy pain, and increasing constipation for two weeks. A cleansing enema at home this morning gave him no relief. His abdomen is tense without rigidity or guarding. It is very tympanitic, and peristalsis seems normal. Rectal negative; no feces in rectum; T 98.6° F.

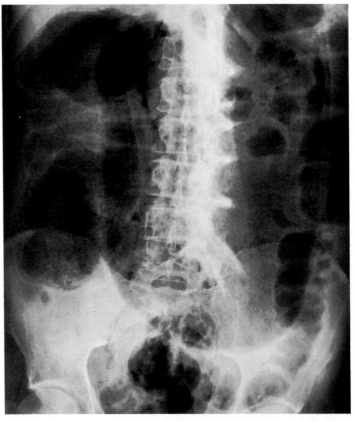

Figure 2–8 Patrick Mahoney

Martha Parks, 31, dressmaker, has had intermittent bouts of pain in her left upper abdomen for three days, severe enough to keep her from finishing a wedding gown promised for Saturday. Her abdomen is distended and tympanitic, with decreased peristalsis and diffuse tenderness, but no guarding or rigidity. T normal.

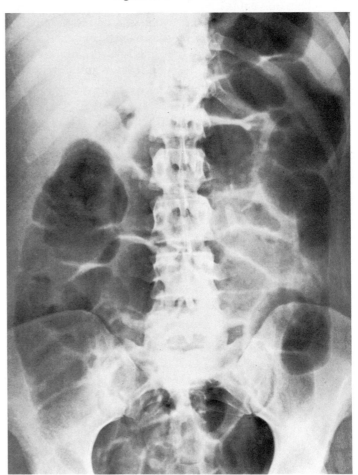

Figure 2–9 Martha Parks

Answers

Mr. Mixter has many distended loops of jejunum, identifiable by their mucosal markings, in the upper and mid abdomen. There are also loops of distended ileum which cross the RLQ obliquely. No gas is seen in any part of the colon and there is no rectal bubble. These are the classic findings in low, small bowel mechanical obstruction with clearing of gas distal to the point of obstruction and dilatation above that point. Mr. Mixter had had an appendectomy 20 years before. At surgery an adhesive band was found at the site causing obstruction near the terminal ileum. He made an excellent recovery.

Mr. Mahoney's story suggests large bowel obstruction. The plain film confirms this, inasmuch as the entire colon is visualized distended with gas. Note that the ascending and transverse colon are very wide in caliber, and that at a point at about mid-descending colon there is a sudden decrease in caliber. A barium enema confirmed the presence of an annular carcinoma at this point narrowing the lumen to less than a centimeter. The wall of the colon above the tumor was markedly thickened. The air in the lower descending colon, sigmoid, and rectum must have been introduced during the enema given at home. A plain film made before the cleansing enema would probably have shown no gas below the point of obstruction and no rectal bubble.

Miss Parks' plain film shows large amounts of gas distending both large and small bowel (follow colon as a "window frame" around from cecum to rectum, and then note the many loops left over, undoubtedly small bowel). This is a roentgen picture consistent with either adynamic ileus *or* low large bowel obstruction in which there is an incompetent ileocecal valve so that gas accumulating in the colon backs up into the small bowel. Miss Parks is young for colon malignancy and the story seems recent and acute. The decreased peristalsis suggests adynamic ileus.

If you noted the large calcific shadow to the left of L3 you will have considered the possibility of a left ureteral calculus. Acute ureteral obstruction is often accompanied by reflex ileus (although it was not in Mrs. Winter in the first group of patients). Overlapping distended loops of bowel make it more difficult to find small calcific shadows along the course of the ureter, and Miss Parks had had no gross hematuria to direct your attention to the possibility of that diagnosis. However, there were red blood cells (RBCs) in the first urinalysis. The excretory urogram (Fig. 2–10) made at 15 minutes shows normal visualization of the right kidney, but absent (or delayed?) visualization of the left. A later film would undoubtedly show the "late white kidney" of acute ureteral obstruction, and the examination should be continued to this point, possibly a matter of several hours. She had ureteroscopy. The calculus was moved back into the renal pelvis. She had extracorporeal lithotripsy (ultrasound crushing) of the calculus into tiny pieces, which she passed over the next couple of days. She finished the wedding gown.

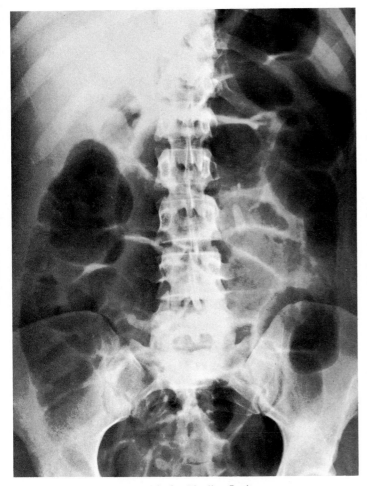

Figure 2-9   Martha Parks

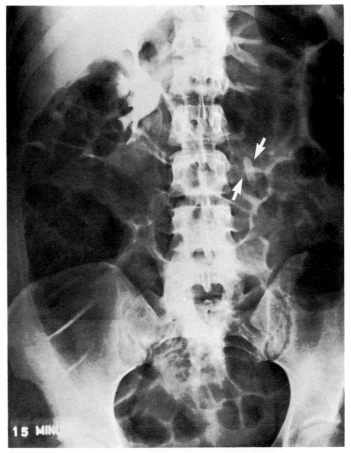

Figure 2-10   Miss Parks, excretory urogram.

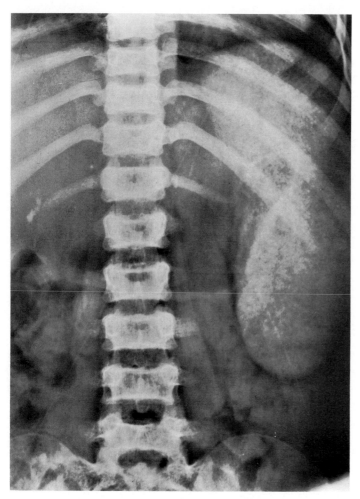

Figure 2–11 Beverley Hamilton

Beverley Hamilton, 18, a black college freshman, is brought to the emergency division in your hospital after collapsing on an airplane. While in flight she had sudden onset of severe upper abdominal pain, nausea, and vomiting. Her upper abdomen is moderately tender but not rigid. The patient is pale, sweats profusely, and complains of headache. She has had three attacks of this sort before. A younger brother is similarly affected. WBC 10,400; hematocrit (Hct) 26. Blood smear shows a normocytic, normochromic anemia with target cells and 10 per cent reticulocytes.

Helen Pickering, 64, typist, comes to you complaining of severe midabdominal cramps and gurgling sounds for several days, worse during the past several hours. She is nauseated but has not vomited. Careful questioning reveals that she has had recent bouts of diarrhea, which she attributes to food intolerance to tomatoes. You find her abdomen distended but soft, with increased peristalsis. T 99.0° F; WBC 9100; Hct 32; reticulocytes 6%.

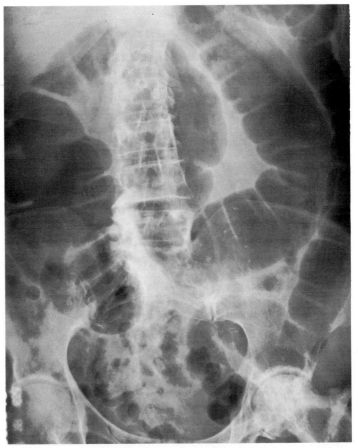

Figure 2–12 Helen Pickering

John Wechsman, 47, stockbroker, has been having crampy epigastric pain for two weeks, relieved, he says, by drinking milk. His abdomen is soft and not distended, and peristalsis is normal. T 98.1° F; WBC 7500; Hct 28; reticulocytes 5%.

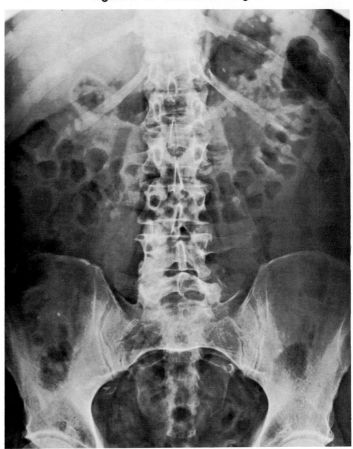

Figure 2–13 John Wechsman

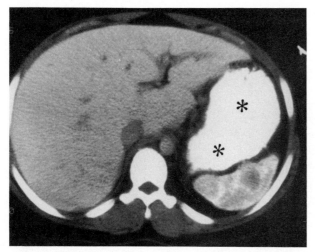

Figure 2–14 Miss Hamilton, CT scan without intravenous contrast. Asterisks are in the contrast-opacified stomach.

Answers

Miss Hamilton proved to have sickle cell anemia in crisis. Tiny calcifications are present in the enlarged spleen, which makes an impression on the stomach. The spleen in young adults with this disease is often (but not always) small and very dense. There are also several small dense concretions in the RUQ that proved to be gallstones, common in the hemolytic anemias, even in childhood. Crises of upper abdominal pain in young black patients, especially when joint pains and anemia are present, must always raise the question of sickle cell disease. The abdominal pain is believed to be due at times to gallstone colic and at others to a variety of ischemic episodes affecting the upper abdominal organs or kidneys, causing hematuria. The flattened, streaky vertebral bodies are also very characteristic. Figure 2–14 is a computed tomogram (CT) through the liver and spleen. Orally ingested contrast material is in the stomach (asterisks). Irregular calcifications are present in the spleen. The liver is normal; unopacified vessels are within the liver.

Miss Pickering's plain film shows distension of large bowel down to a point in midsigmoid and no rectal bubble. This finding, together with her age and story, suggests the possibility of carcinoma of the sigmoid colon. This was confirmed by barium enema (Fig. 2–15). The hemogram was that of chronic blood loss and the stools were guaiac-positive. At surgery her annular sigmoid carcinoma was found not to extend to regional nodes or liver and she was alive ten years later.

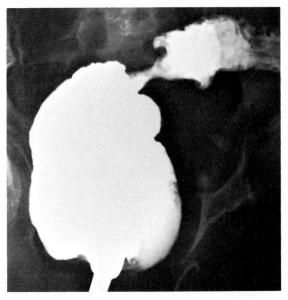

Figure 2–15   Miss Pickering, barium enema.

Mr. Wechsman's story suggests the possibility of a peptic ulcer. His plain film is entirely normal, but his gastrointestinal study showed the presence of an active ulcer in a moderately deformed duodenal bulb (Fig. 2–16). His hemogram was consistent with acute blood loss and his stools were guaiac-positive although he could not remember noting dark stools. He responded fairly well to an ulcer regimen, but his hematocrit values tended to fluctuate with the Dow-Jones averages.

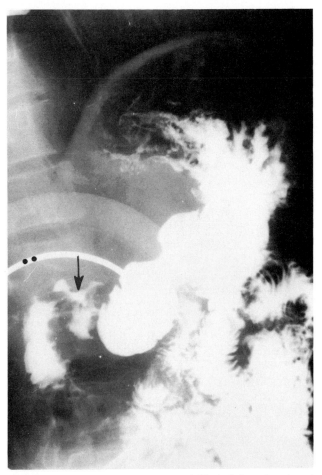

Figure 2–16   Mr. Wechsman, spot film of the duodenal bulb. The metallic rim (twin black dots) is part of a compression balloon. Arrow points to ulcer crater.

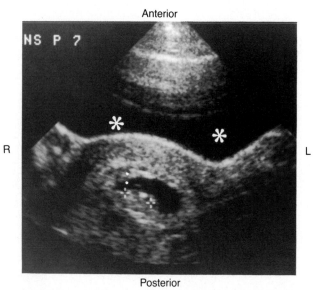

Anterior

Posterior

Figure 2–17 Mary Cook, pelvic ultrasound. Asterisks are in the urinary bladder.

Mary Cook, 28, gravida III, para II, comes to the obstetric clinic with a history of two missed periods and frequent RUQ pain after heavy meals.

Norma Palizzio, 25, x-ray file clerk, is brought to emergency because of acute abdominal pain. On examination, there is an exquisitely tender suprapubic mass present. Hct 36; WBC 9200; T 99.7° F; pulse (P) 100; respiration (R) 20. Her serum human chorionic gonadotropin level did *not* suggest pregnancy.

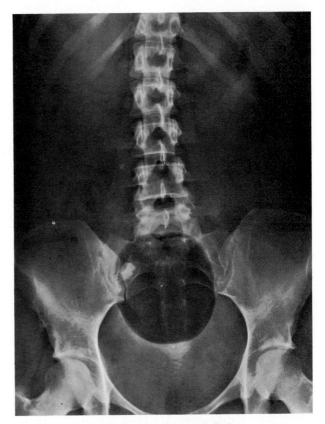

Figure 2–18 Norma Palizzio

Violet McComber, 18, married, no children, is admitted after the sudden onset of abdominal pain and vomiting. The pain started in the epigastrium, but has become more severe as it moved down into the RLQ. She has missed two periods. On both pelvic and rectal examination there is a boggy ill-defined tender mass present to the right of a normal uterus. The abdomen is tense and diffusely tender with RLQ guarding. Hct 28; WBC 8000; T 98.1° F; P 90; R 18.

Figure 2–19 Violet McComber, pelvic ultrasound. Asterisk indicates the bladder; arrows point to the uterus.

Answers

Mrs. Cook is multiparous with two separate significant complaints: (1) missed period implying pregnancy, and (2) postprandial RUQ pain suggestive of gallbladder disease, a frequent occurrence in multiparous women. Ultrasound is the best examination for the evaluation of suspected pregnancy and gallbladder disease. Figure 2–17 is a pelvic ultrasound that shows an intrauterine gestational sac with an identifiable fetal pole (between marks). The measurement of this tiny fetal pole corresponds to a gestational age of 7.3 weeks. Asterisks are in the urinary bladder. Figure 2–20 is an ultrasound of Mrs. Cook's gallbladder. The echogenic focus with acoustic shadowing represents a gallstone. Figure 2–21 is a normal gallbladder ultrasound for comparison.

Miss Palizzio's acute symptoms were due to a twisted ovarian dermoid cyst. The strikingly round, very radiolucent structure overlying the sacrum cannot be air in the bowel, and, besides, it contains what appears to be a tooth. Fatty grumous material in dermoid cysts is usually radiolucent compared with surrounding structures of water density. Emergency surgery showed a bluish, strangulated left cystic ovary, which was resected. The right ovary was normal.

Mrs. McComber's symptoms of severe pelvo-abdominal pain and missed periods should alert you to a first-trimester obstetric emergency: ectopic pregnancy. Figure 2–19 is an emergency pelvic ultrasound of the pelvis that shows a right-sided ectopic gestation. A well-defined gestational sac with a fetal pole (between markers) is in the right adnexa—adjacent to the uterus. Arrows point to the uterus; asterisk is in the urinary bladder. An ectopic pregnancy was found at exploratory laparoscopy in the right fallopian tube. Because of prompt diagnosis, this ectopic pregnancy has not ruptured.

Figure 2–22 is a CT demonstration of a massive hemoperitoneum in another female patient who had a splenic rupture following a motor vehicle accident. Notice the uterus and the broad ligaments. These structures are exceptionally well demonstrated because of the large amount of peritoneal fluid.

When an ectopic pregnancy ruptures, massive life-threatening hemoperitoneum may occur as with a ruptured spleen. A suspected ectopic pregnancy is an emergency.

Figure 2–23 is an ultrasound of another pregnant patient. What is your diagnosis? (See answer at bottom of page.)

Figure 2–24 is magnetic resonance imaging (MRI) on a pregnant patient. She was not known to be pregnant prior to the examination, which was done to rule out aseptic necrosis of the hips. Although MRI is not believed to be harmful to the fetus, its safety has not been tested to this point. Notice the fetus is in the breech presentation.

Early twin gestation.

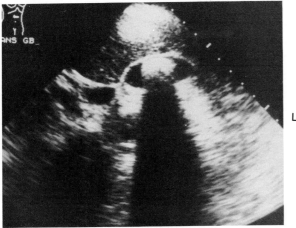

Anterior

R   L

Posterior

Figure 2–20   Mrs. Cook, gallbladder ultrasound.

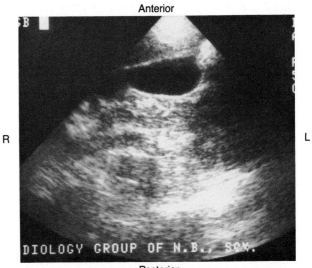

Anterior

R   L

Posterior

Figure 2–21   Normal gallbladder ultrasound.

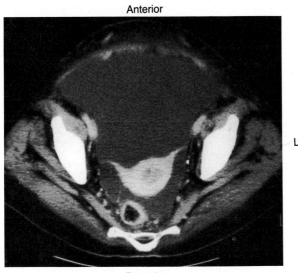

Anterior

R   L

Posterior

Figure 2–22   CT scan.

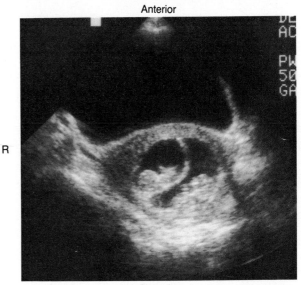

Anterior

R   L

Posterior

Figure 2–23   Ultrasound in pregnancy.

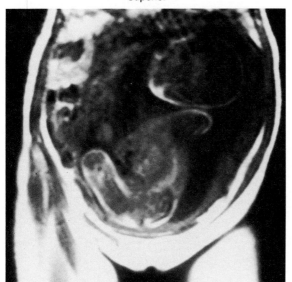

Superior

R   L

Inferior

Figure 2–24   MRI in pregnancy.

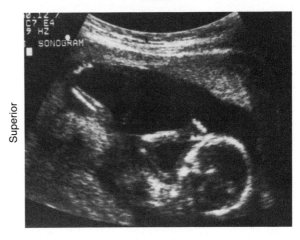

Anterior

Superior   Inferior

Posterior

Figure 2–25   "What a headache!" is the impression you get from this obstetrical ultrasound of a fetus of about 22 to 23 weeks.

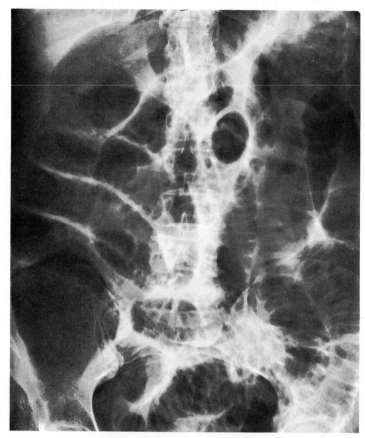

Figure 2–26 Barbara Karch

Barbara Karch, 60, lives alone with her five cats. She comes to clinic complaining of constipation and abdominal swelling for four weeks. She has had no bleeding of any sort and has not lost weight. She has had one or two bouts of loose stools, however, and noticed mucus in them. Her abdomen is quite distended and tympanitic but without any guarding or rigidity. Rectal examination is negative. No feces in the rectum. Bowel sounds are active and normal. TPR normal; Hct 32.

Phyllis Abele, 40, has been paraplegic since a skiing accident ten years ago. She is in the hospital on the medical service recovering from pneumonia. You are asked to see her on a surgical consultation because of constipation and abdominal distension for two days with generalized abdominal pain. Her abdomen is tympanitic and diffusely tender and bowel sounds are decreased. T 100° F; P 88; R 22; Hct 38; WBC 12,000.

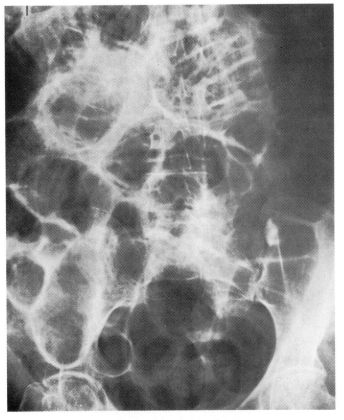

Figure 2–27 Phyllis Abele

Robert McCandliss, 57, has been bedridden for many years in a nursing home with multiple sclerosis and paraplegia. He is brought to the hospital by ambulance because he has been complaining of abdominal pain, crampy in character, for one week, and he had his last bowel movement (BM) three days ago. His abdomen is grossly distended and tympanitic, with moderate discomfort on palpation but no guarding or rigidity. Rectal negative; TPR normal; Hct 38.

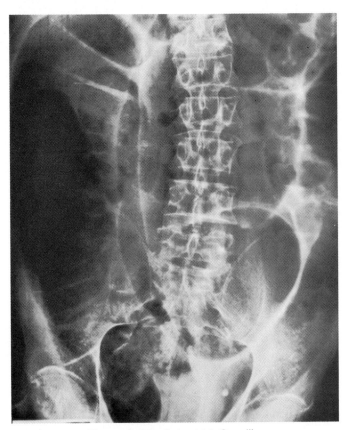

Figure 2–28 Robert McCandliss

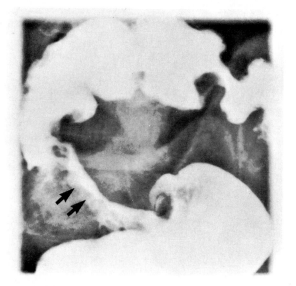

Figure 2–29 Miss Karch, barium enema. Arrows point to irregularly narrowed sigmoid.

Answers

Miss Karch's plain film shows marked gaseous distension of both large and small bowel. She does not have a silent abdomen, and her story suggests low large bowel obstruction; the film would confirm such a tentative diagnosis if one supposes the ileocecal valve to be incompetent. Barium enema was done and showed a long segment of narrowed sigmoid just above the rectosigmoid junction (Fig. 2–29), which was resected and proved to be carcinoma. (Note: this lesion was easily visualized by endoscopy but not felt on rectal examination.) You may wonder why a barium enema was necessary after the lesion was visualized by sigmoidoscopy and the diagnosis of carcinoma suspected. The sigmoidoscopic appearance of colon lesions, whether inflammatory or neoplastic, is frequently confusing, whereas the roentgen appearance with barium may be classic. It is also desirable to delineate the full extent of the lesion as a guide to the surgical approach.

Miss Abele also has distended loops of large and small bowel. Her hemiplegia, recent febrile illness in bed in the hospital, and silent abdomen all suggest that adynamic ileus is a good deal more probable than mechanical obstruction as a cause of her distension and constipation. It was easy to make sure, however: Figure 2–30 is her barium enema and shows ready passage of barium to the cecum and terminal ileum, excluding large bowel obstruction.

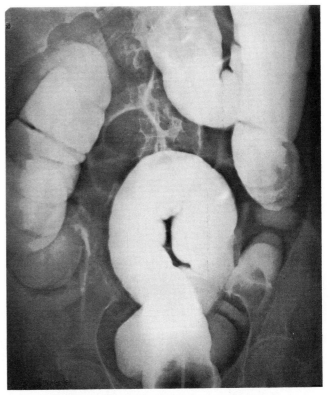

Figure 2–30   Miss Abele, barium enema.

Mr. McCandliss' plain film shows widely distended bowel, which is clearly colon. There is very little gas in the small bowel and no rectal bubble. Some sort of low large bowel obstruction is implied. Centrally located colon, dramatically dilated to this extent, should at once suggest sigmoid volvulus. Again the barium enema makes the diagnosis: A beak-like twist of sigmoid is pathognomonic of sigmoid volvulus (Fig. 2–31). Either the sigmoidoscopic examination or the barium enema may prove therapeutic in decompressing the twisted loop.

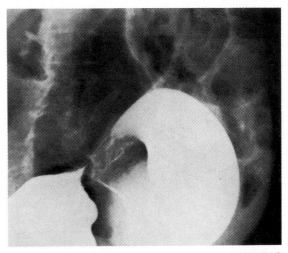

Figure 2–31   Mr. McCandliss, barium enema (detail). Only a limited barium study is done. No attempt is made to fill further than the twisted segment.

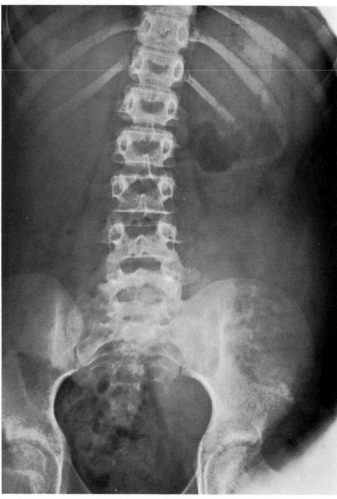

Figure 2–32 Bobby Phillips

Bobby Phillips, 12, is just getting over a bad cold, but has been complaining increasingly of pain in his abdomen. There is tenderness and guarding in the LLQ, his temperature is 104° F, and WBC 18,000. He lies with his left thigh flexed. Rectal examination elicits tenderness on the left.

Arabella Sniffen, 28, has been visiting an aunt in town. She comes to emergency on a Saturday night complaining of constant costovertebral angle (CVA) pain and tenderness, with fever (100.9° F), and says she has had similar attacks before. You find CVA pain on percussion, and the right kidney seems tender. There are no other abdominal findings. WBC 14,000.

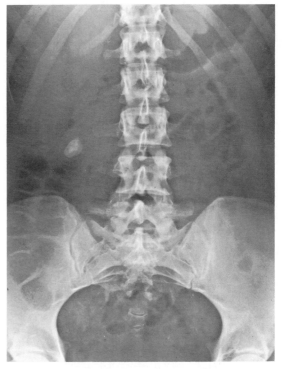

Figure 2–33 Arabella Sniffen

Stephen Borden, 38, an unemployed, homeless alcoholic, has been found by the police, drunk and groaning, in the doorway of a condemned building. He is "ill-kempt" (with scabies and body lice) and "uncooperative" (noisy, truculent, and combative, resisting both questioning and examination). Physical exam, insofar as it can be carried out, is negative except for the abdomen, which seems to be tender and rigid in both upper quadrants. Rectal, a losing battle, is not done; T 102.2° F; P 100; R 30; WBC 16,000.

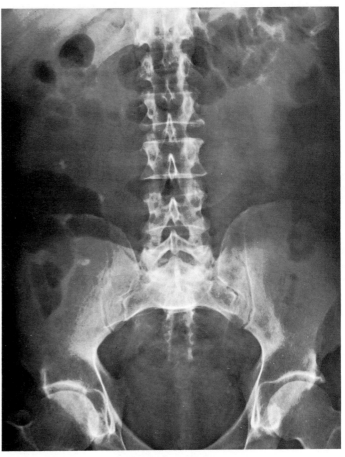

Figure 2–34 Stephen Borden

Answers

Bobby Phillips' plain film helps you because it confirms the physical findings suggesting an acute inflammatory process in the LLQ. Note that the normal tip of spleen, stomach shadow, lower pole of left kidney, outline of right kidney, and entire right psoas margin may be identified. The left psoas shadow ends abruptly opposite L3. Bowel gas is swept out of the LLQ by a soft tissue mass that is ill-defined except where it projects into the bowl of the pelvis. This interface running sharply across from the left side of the sacrum toward the left acetabulum is altogether abnormal and must be accounted for. The disappearance of psoas margin indicates edema of the fat in the psoas sheath. An abscess in the psoas sheath will extend inferiorly and present as a pelvic mass, as it does here. Note scoliosis with concavity to the left and rows of bubbles of "uncontained" gas overlying the left iliac wing and obviously not inside gut.

Both CT scanning and sonography were considered at this point. Sonography was elected, however, to avoid irradiation of a young patient. The sonogram of the abdomen confirmed the presence of a predominantly fluid collection in the retroperitoneum. Percutaneous drainage of the large psoas abscess was carried out.

Miss Sniffen has normal gas shadows locating the stomach, small bowel, and right colon. The upper pole of the left kidney is seen, but the right is impossible to outline. A large calcific shadow to the right of L3 could be either in the right kidney or in the gall bladder. The CVA tenderness suggests kidney disease, and you find her urine loaded with pus and RBCs. An excretory urogram (Fig. 2–35) shows the stone lying in a dilated and eroded calyx in the lower pole of the right kidney. The dilated upper pole calices in both kidneys come so close to the kidney margins that there must be only a very thin functioning parenchyma remaining. These findings are classic for chronic pyelonephritis. Figure 2–36 is an excretory study made six years later and shows further shrinkage of the right kidney.

Figure 2–37 is another patient with pyelonephritic change much less severe than that seen in Miss Sniffen. The changes to note are dilated and blunted calices and thinned kidney parenchyma.

Mr. Borden's plain film is entirely normal. His tenderness and rigidity proved to be reflex and were related to his bilateral lower lobe pneumonia (juxtadiaphragmatic), which was not diagnosed until six hours after admission. (For a discussion and clear indications to help in avoiding this mistake, see pages 85 and 193 in Cope, Z.: *The Early Diagnosis of The Acute Abdomen*, 13th Ed., Oxford University Press.)

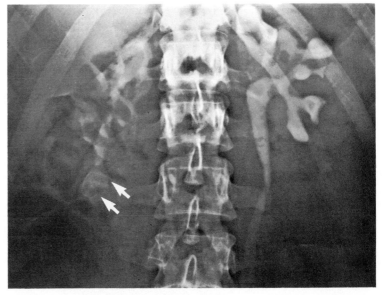

Figure 2–35

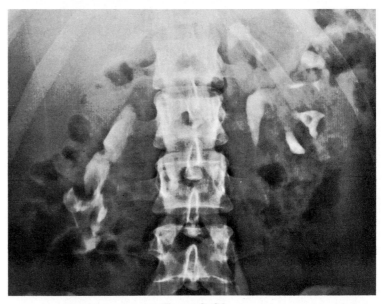

Figure 2–36

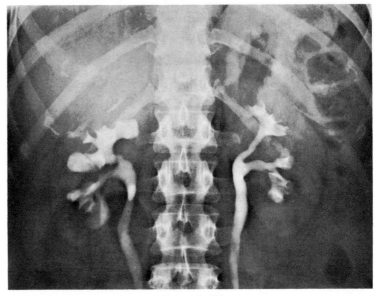

Figure 2–37

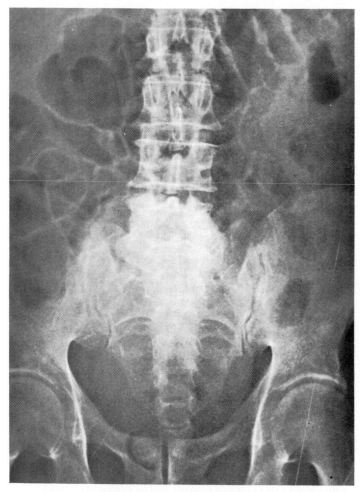

Figure 2—38 Robert Mandelis

Robert Mandelis, 71, retired Latvian carpenter, is brought to the hospital confused, disoriented, and in some sort of pain that he cannot define for you because of his poor command of English. However, he holds his lower abdomen with both hands and moans. TPR normal. You find a tender, smooth, cystic, lower abdominal midline mass extending up to the umbilicus. There is no guarding. Rectal examination elicits some generalized painful response and the prostate is enlarged.

Darrell Krump, a 47-year-old tax attorney, was brought to the emergency room by his partner after he complained of severe lower abdominal pain shortly after lunch. He has not felt well over the last couple of days and thought he had some fever. On physical examination he had exquisite RLQ tenderness and peritoneal signs. He had a WBC of 17,000. He sounds as if he has appendicitis. He gives you a history of inflammatory bowel disease while he was in college. To confirm your impression, you order a supine abdominal film and an abdominal CT.

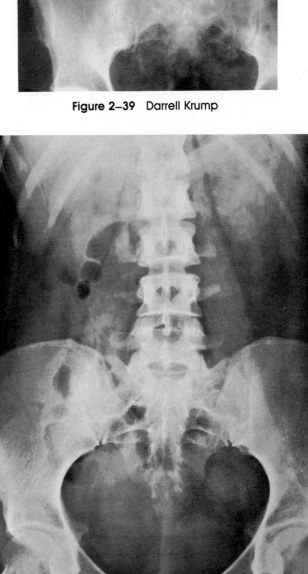

Figure 2–39 Darrell Krump

Lavinia Duane, 36, sales clerk, has been admitted because of vaginal spotting and RLQ pain for one week. The patient says she has missed one period but insists she is not pregnant. She says she has been treated in gynecology clinic for a "pus tube." Nobody can find her record in the record room. The abdominal examination is not remarkable, but the rectal shows the presence of a tender, boggy mass on the right. T 98.2° F; P 85; R 16; blood pressure (BP) 120/70. The emergency room resident orders a plain film (Fig. 2–40).

Figure 2–40 Lavinia Duane

Melinda Moss, 28, mother of three, one week following elective tubal ligation developed severe lower abdominal pain and high fever. Her Hct was 21; WBC 22,000. On physical examination she had exquisite suprapubic tenderness and a palpable adnexal mass.

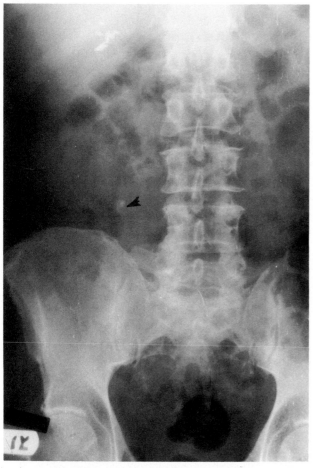

Figure 2-41   Mr. Darrell Krump

Answers

Mr. Mandelis' plain film shows a water density soft tissue mass rising out of the pelvis. Note that there is no tangentially seen perivesical fat line present separating it from the usual bladder shadow. This mass proved to be the bladder itself, obstructed by the enlarged prostate, and it completely disappeared when the patient was catheterized. The crescentic lucent shadow over the right pubis is air around a solid fecal bolus in the rectum; the enlarged prostate would not be seen, as it is the same density as urine in the bladder.

Figure 2-39 demonstrates few small air bubbles in the RLQ (arrows). Figure 2-41 arrowhead points to a faintly calcified appendolith. Figure 2-42 is a section from his abdominal CT scan, which at the level of the pelvic inlet on the right shows an abnormality: air bubbles in an abscess (black arrows). He had exploratory laparotomy during which a gangrenous perforated appendix was found with an abscess cavity.

Anterior

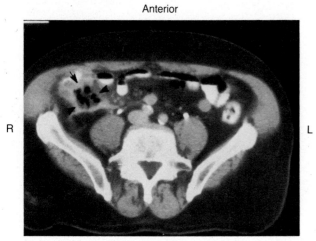

Posterior

Figure 2-42   Mr. Krump

In retrospect the emergency resident should have requested sonography as the initial diagnostic study in *Miss Duane*. The sonogram would certainly have shown a complex pelvic mass on the right side and possibly a gestational sac, which would clinch the diagnosis. In any case the sonogram was not done.

Miss Duane's record did show an earlier series of visits to gynecology clinic for acute and chronic pelvic inflammatory disease, and a right adnexal mass was described. The plain film shows (Fig. 2–40) a mass consistent with this finding; note that it is seen to be separated from the bladder by the perivesical fat line. The patient's Hct, 38 on admission, subsequently fell to 32 and she appeared to be in incipient shock with a BP of 80/60. Emergency laparotomy showed 1000 ml of free blood in the peritoneal cavity and a ruptured tubal pregnancy adherent to the right adnexal mass. Notice how the most appropriate examination for a suspected clinical problem can help you make an immediate diagnosis. Figure 2–19 shows an ectopic pregnancy on pelvic ultrasound; the plain abdominal film, Figure 2–40, helps you very little.

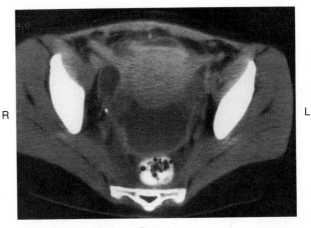

Anterior

Posterior

Figure 2–43 Melinda Moss. Identify iliac bones, coccyx, rectum, and uterus.

Mrs. Moss had CT scan of the pelvis (Fig. 2–43), which shows two collections in the pelvis. Where is the larger collection in relation to the uterus? Figure 2–44 is a slightly lower CT section of the pelvis on Mrs. Moss, which shows the superior aspect of the urinary bladder and both ureters (small round contrast-filled structures). The larger collection (asterisk) is posterior to the uterus (black arrow is in utero). The smaller collection is in the right adnexa (smaller asterisk). After being placed on large doses of antibiotics, she had transvaginal catheter drainage by the radiologist. The material obtained was pus and old blood. She required several more drainage catheters over the next two to three weeks. Several weeks later she was back to her usual activities.

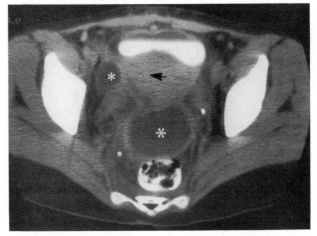

Figure 2–44 Mrs. Moss. CT of pelvis at a slightly lower level shows contrast-filled urinary bladder just anterior to the uterus (arrow in uterus). Asterisks designate abscess collections. Notice the opaque dots are contrast-filled ureters.

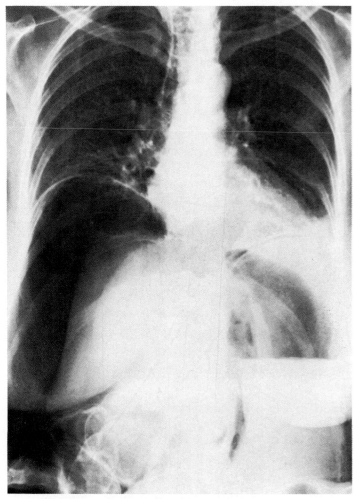

Figure 2–45 Barbara Martin

Barbara Martin, 48, customer at Park's Department Store, fainted while trying on some gloves. Brought in by ambulance, she is now conscious, pale, and anxious, and complains of pain on top of her right shoulder. She vomited on her way to the hospital, and examination shows her upper abdomen to be rigid. T 98.1° F; P 110; R 32; BP 110/90.

Ruth Wieland, 44, buyer in the infant's wear division at Park's, fainted after complaining all morning of epigastric and left shoulder pain. She is sweating and her T is 98.1° F, P 100, BP 90/60. You find epigastric tenderness and guarding.

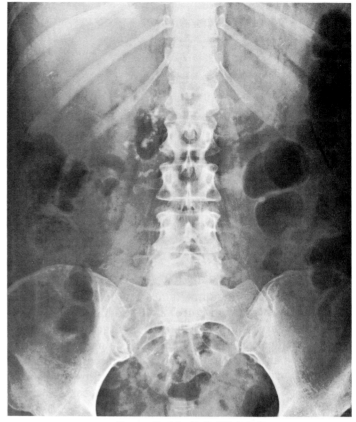

Figure 2–46 Ruth Wieland

Martha Infelder, 21, shoplifter at Park's, fainted during her usual tour of duty and is brought to emergency by Mr. Park himself who happened to be in the store. The patient complained of pain on top of her left shoulder on regaining consciousness and says she is just recovering from infectious mononucleosis. T 96.1° F; P 110; R 26; BP 90/60.

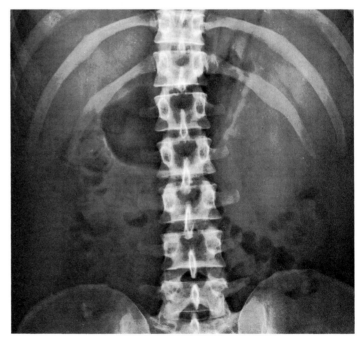

Figure 2–47 Martha Infelder

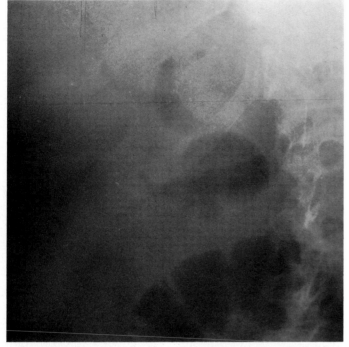

Figure 2–55 Air in the biliary tree; branching black streaks high over the liver in another patient with gallstone obstruction.

Answers

Miss Winwood's plain film shows several loops of distended midabdominal small bowel (jejunum) and no "window frame" of colon to be identified by its air or fecal content. Colon and jejunum, when distended to the same caliber, may generally be distinguished from each other by the *periodicity* of crosswise mucosal ridges (i.e., the number of ridges per running inch). Colon will have fewer ridges and, of course, haustra do not usually cross the bowel from one side to the other as the valvulae conniventes in the jejunum do. The loops in Figure 2–52 are all small bowel, and the roentgen diagnosis is advanced mechanical small bowel obstruction with clearing of the colon. At surgery a large solitary gallstone was found impacted in a loop of ileum. It cannot be seen on the plain film.

This is therefore *gallstone obstruction,* a much better term than "gallstone ileus" because the mechanical nature of the obstruction is clear. Branching black streaks of air in the biliary tree are often seen over the liver and indicate a spontaneous internal fistula between the gallbladder and the second portion of the duodenum where the stone has been passed into the bowel (Fig. 2–55).

Mrs. Gomez' plain film confirms the rather clear clinical impression of mechanical small bowel obstruction in that there are widely distended jejunal and ileal loops and little or no air remaining in the colon. An erect film (Fig. 2–56) shows the classic "dynamic (or hairpin) loops" of mechanical obstruction. Note that it is easy to pick out two fluid-air interfaces belonging to the same loop and that they are at *different* levels. Hairpin loops are not always present in mechanical obstruction and are not essential to the diagnosis. When they are present, the diagnosis is reinforced. Mrs. Gomez was found to have adhesions at the site of the recent surgery.

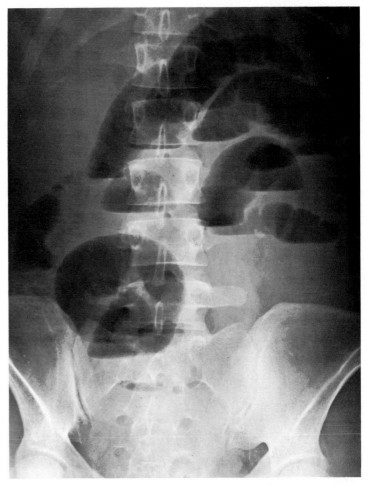

Figure 2–56 Mrs. Gomez, erect film.

Miss Feathers' abdominal plain film shows nothing abnormal. Tips of spleen and liver can be seen. Her psoas muscle shadows are clear and gas is scattered through stomach and colon normally. Ultimately this patient proved to have temporal lobe epilepsy. The electroencephalogram (EEG) demonstrated a consistently abnormal temporal lobe discharge, accentuated during sleep. Abdominal pain is not at all rare as a manifestation of epilepsy, either as its aura or as its sole symptom. More careful history disclosed that this patient had on occasion had lapses of consciousness and "automatic behavior" associated with the epigastric pain. That the attacks frequently occurred at times of emotional stress had raised the question of hysteria. Attacks were controlled on anticonvulsant regimen.

THREE PATIENTS WITH NAUSEA, VOMITING, AND ABDOMINAL PAIN BUT DECREASED PERISTALSIS

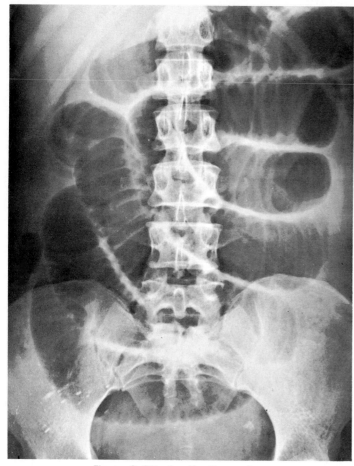

Figure 2–57   Agatha Ponsonby

Agatha Ponsonby, 44, receptionist, was well until five days ago when she developed crampy lower abdominal pain, nausea, and vomiting. Her abdomen is distended but not rigid, although there is guarding over the lower abdomen. The patient looks exhausted. Peristalsis is limited to rare sounds, which you find so hard to believe in view of the plain film that you listen carefully several times. Rectal reveals a tender pelvic mass. T 100° F; P 100; WBC 20,900.

Euphemia Partridge, 37, a Christian Science reader, has had nausea, vomiting, and abdominal distension for six days and has only reluctantly agreed to be brought to the hospital by her landlady. She appears very dehydrated. The abdomen is quite distended but not as tympanitic as you expect it to be and not rigid. There are no bowel sounds at all. T 100.9° F; P 110.

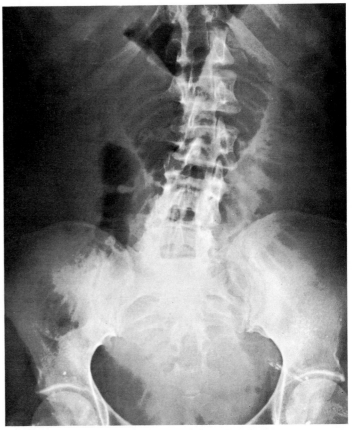

Figure 2-58 Euphemia Partridge

Maxine Tilley, 38, librarian, had a hysterectomy two days ago, and is seen because of complaints of crampy abdominal pain that have fluctuated in severity for 36 hours. She is nauseated and has vomited once. The abdomen is very distended but she is passing flatus. Peristalsis is decreased to absent. T 99° F; P 86.

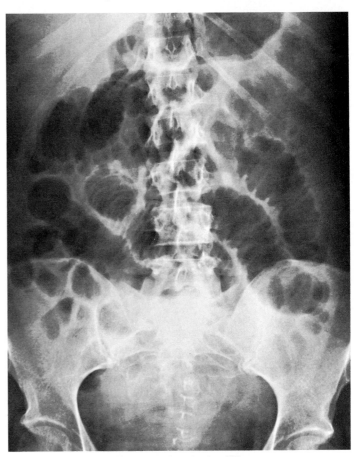

Figure 2-59 Maxine Tilley

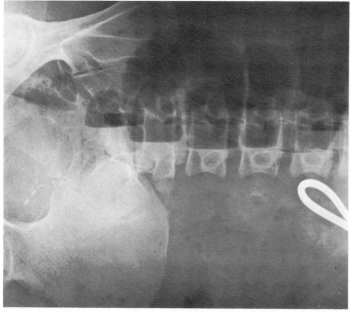

Figure 2–60 Mrs. Ponsonby, decubitus film.

Answers

Mrs. Ponsonby's plain film shows distended jejunal loops. A roentgen impression of mechanical small bowel obstruction is inescapable, and in sharp conflict with the finding of decreased peristalsis . . . *except* in patients in advanced stages of obstruction when the bowel may decompensate. Her decubitus film (Fig. 2–60) shows hairpin loops, but their fluid levels are virtually at the same level indicating the absence of peristaltic forward rushes. (Paralytic ileus may also develop when this kind of delay results in perforation of the obstructed bowel and peritonitis.) At surgery a loop of ileum was found adherent to an inflammatory right adnexal mass.

Miss Partridge has distended loops of jejunum and little or no air in colon, but her abdominal plain film is surprisingly dense. This is explained when the decubitus film is examined (Fig. 2–61). Relatively little air and a great deal of fluid are filling her obstructed loops of small bowel. Some of these are indicated only by strings of bubbles caught between the mucosal ridges. The heavy fluid-filled parts of the loops merge their shadows together and are responsible for the generally increased density of this film. This patient is dehydrated into her bowel and in far worse condition preoperatively than the preceding patient, since her electrolytes must be seriously deranged. Absence of peristalsis here again indicates either bowel decompensation, ileus, or peritonitis. Vascular insufficiency must also be considered in the presence of fluid-filled loops. Prompt surgery and freeing of a knuckle of ileum in an unsuspected femoral hernia did not save this patient, who died on the operating table.

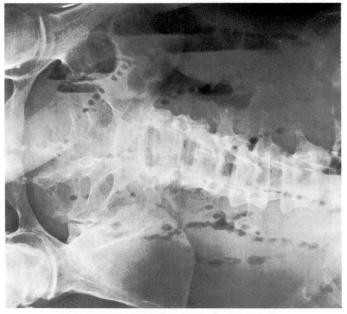

Figure 2–61   Miss Partridge, decubitus film.

Mrs. Tilley has midline metallic stay sutures and distended stomach, jejunum, and ileum. It is hard to be certain whether or not there is air in colon. Here it is vital to make a differential diagnosis between postoperative obstruction and postoperative ileus; the former will require surgery, whereas the latter might be treated conservatively. The story suggests ileus, but the plain film is equivocal. A decubitus film with the right side up (Fig. 2–62) shows definite air in the colon and reinforces the impression that this patient has paralytic ileus and may be watched. A nasogastric tube was passed and the patient recovered without having her incision taken down.

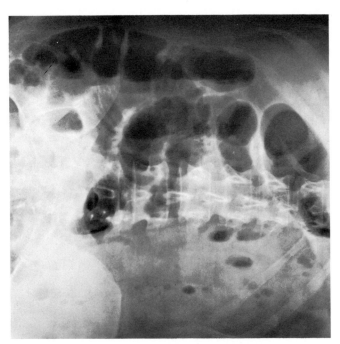

Figure 2–62   Mrs. Tilley, decubitus film.

All three patients have been filmed lying on the left side facing you, and a horizontal beam has been used: the left lateral decubitus.

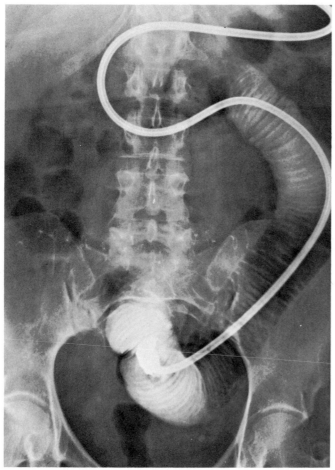

Figure 2–63

Answers (*Continued*)

The following are other maneuvers that may prove helpful in differentiating paralytic ileus from mechanical obstruction.

Figure 2–63 shows a postoperative patient who has a single, long, distended loop of jejunum. A Miller-Abbott (MA) tube has been passed and the tip has arrested at the point of mechanical obstruction. A small amount of dilute contrast substance (barium is often used) is injected through the tube, and the fact of complete obstruction is established. At times some information as to the nature of the obstructing lesion may also be obtained by this type of study.

Figure 2–64 shows a patient in whom mechanical obstruction was proved to be absent when contrast material passed through into the colon. This was one day after hysterectomy, and the patient developed abdominal distension with intermittent cramps and normal peristalsis. The plain film showed some air in both small bowel and colon. Such a roentgen picture can be equivocal, representing either ileus or incomplete (or early) mechanical obstruction. This procedure of introducing barium through an MA tube should not be undertaken if there is a possibility of low large bowel obstruction; in that event a barium enema should be done before the procedure shown here.

When the diagnosis of small bowel obstruction is uncertain, both clinically and from the roentgenograms, following the patient closely, clinically, and with subsequent abdominal films can suggest obstruction with more certainty.

Recent evidence exists that CT of the abdomen may best define the point of obstruction.

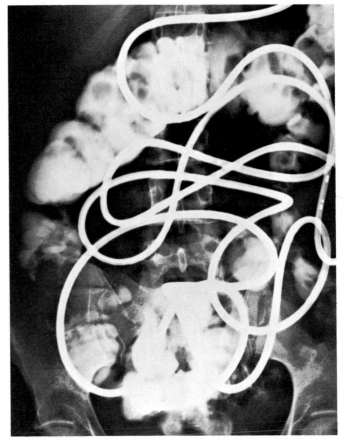

Figure 2–64

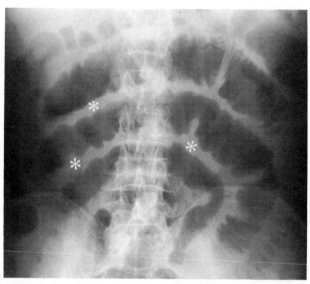

Figure 2–65 Felicity Frisk

Felicity Frisk, 65, librarian at the local high school, arrives at the hospital complaining of gradually increasing abdominal girth that makes it difficult for her to bend and stoop as she goes about her duties. She also complains of constipation. She has been gaining weight for some time.

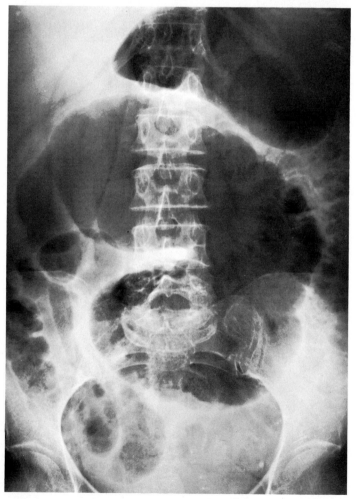

Figure 2–66 Eleana Pogsdale

Eleana Pogsdale, 62, a widow living at one of the Leisure World villages for senior citizens, is brought to the emergency division complaining of a tensely distended abdomen. During the week since the distension began she has had some relief from repeated enemas. Her past history is unremarkable except for mild hypertension.

James Groat, 56, taxi driver, comes to clinic because of increasing abdominal distension, occasional crampy pains and constipation unusual for him. He is a testy, impatient, plethoric man whom you remember having been in clinic last week, but who left before he could be seen. His chart shows he was studied three years ago after an episode of chest pain; he was found to have hypertension but no electrocardiographic (ECG) abnormality suggesting myocardial infarction. He has recently lost 15 pounds and has no appetite.

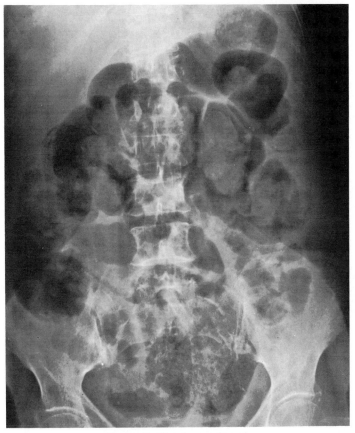

Figure 2–67 James Groat

Answers

Mrs. Frisk's supine abdominal film shows numerous small bowel loops in the midabdomen that are separated from one another by fluid (asterisks). This is a helpful plain film finding suggestive of ascites. Often ascites is difficult to ascertain on plain films. Ultrasound and CT can detect minuscule amounts of fluid in the peritoneal cavity.

Mrs. Pogsdale had surgery the same evening for a cecal volvulus that had been recognized from the plain film and confirmed by barium enema. Note that the stomach is seen high in the LUQ, that the large central gas shadow *looks like* large bowel, and that the rest of the colon is empty. There is no identifiable cecal shadow in the RLQ. The gas shadows on the left side of the abdomen are loops of dilated jejunum pushed to the left by the acutely distended cecum. The barium enema showed free passage of barium through a collapsed colon to a beak-like twist that prevented filling of the cecum. At surgery the cecum was greatly distended, with several small gangrenous areas but no actual perforation. The patient made an excellent recovery.

Mr. Groat's plain film shows colon distended with air and fecal material. On physical examination his rectum was empty. The story suggests large bowel obstruction. Barium enema showed an annular obstructing carcinoma in the descending colon, which was successfully resected.

During his convalescence Mr. Groat had another episode suggesting myocardial ischemia. In patients with evidence of cardiovascular disease and any sort of abdominal symptoms, one must always consider the possibility of abdominal vascular disease. However, the acute clinical symptoms of abdominal angina or of mesenteric thrombosis or infarction are usually not difficult to differentiate from the gradually obstructing low colonic lesion. Barium enema is an excellent method of demonstrating a colonic lesion. To be sure, patients with vascular occlusive disease of the intestine are generally much sicker than Mr. Groat was.

Other Causes of Abdominal Distension

Figure 2–68 shows distension of both large and small bowel in a patient with chronic constipation. Note the speckled midline rectal bubble filled with feces rather than with air. The patient was elderly and bedridden; constipation was of long standing and there were no acute symptoms.

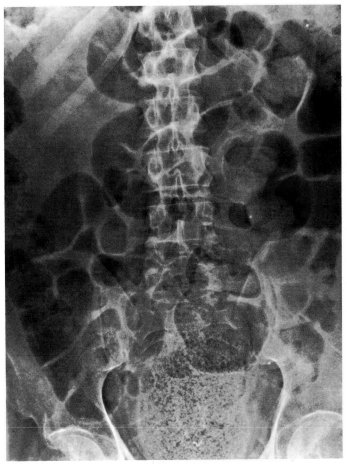

Figure 2–68

Figure 2–69 shows abdominal distension due to a distended stomach. This was a patient with impending diabetic coma and gastroparesis diabeticorum. Other causes of gastric outlet obstruction include ulcer disease, acute pancreatitis, duodenal mass secondary to a hematoma and neoplasm.

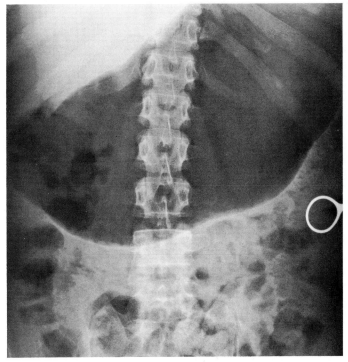

Figure 2–69

TWO PATIENTS WHO PRESENTED WITH DISTENSION, ABDOMINAL PAIN, AND RIGIDITY AND WHOSE PLAIN FILMS INDICATE THE DIAGNOSIS

Dorchas Mayling, 62, thought by her family to be a professional invalid, has a 42-year history of varied gastrointestinal complaints. She had her first laparotomy at age 23 for "intestinal obstruction" and since then has had frequent episodes of vomiting, diarrhea, distension, and migratory abdominal pain. One week ago her abdomen became distended and today she vomited several times. Examination shows her abdomen to be distended and tense, tender, and rigid. There are no bowel sounds. (Note: The correct diagnosis was proposed preoperatively from the supine and erect plain films, Figures 2–70 and 2–71, respectively.)

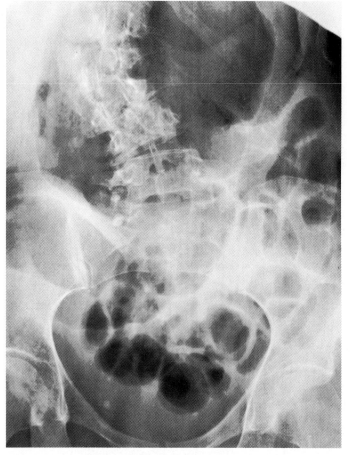

Figure 2–70   Dorchas Mayling

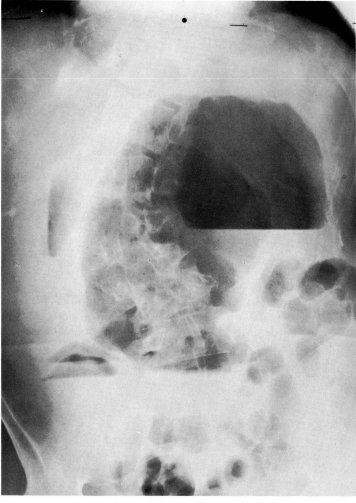

Figure 2–71   Miss Mayling, upright film.

H. Hawk Handsaw, 49, detective, is admitted with a story of ten days of mild, crampy lower abdominal pain with some diarrhea. He vomited this morning. He now has a distended, tense, rigid, silent abdomen. (Note: The correct diagnosis was proposed from the supine plain film.)

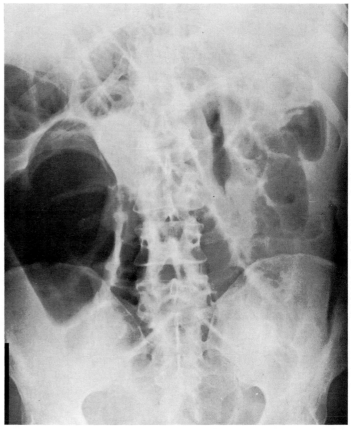

Figure 2–72 H. Hawk Handsaw

Answers

Miss Mayling's supine plain film (Fig. 2–70) shows loops of distended small bowel in mid- and left abdomen but no midline rectal bubble. In the upper midabdomen there is a widely distended, gas-filled structure that *might* be stomach. It is hard to decide how much air-filled colon is present. Figure 2–71, the upright film including the diaphragm, shows the large, gas-filled, central structure set down and separated from the left diaphragm. Stomach almost never does this, being fixed at the cardia. A tentative preoperative diagnosis of cecal volvulus was made, and, because of clinical findings suggesting perforation and impending peritonitis, a laparotomy was performed without waiting for either decubitus films (for free air?) or a barium enema (confirming the diagnosis of volvulus). Multiple adhesions and a cecal volvulus with gangrene, perforation, and diffuse peritoneal soilage were encountered.

Mr. Handsaw's supine plain film shows distended large and small bowel. The intern thought he might have a perforated viscus and peritonitis and requested an erect film (Fig. 2–73). The diaphragm was not included, unfortunately, so that although there are many fluid- and air-filled loops, no additional information is really obtained. The patient was refilmed standing (Fig. 2–74) and shows the very small amount of free air underneath the diaphragms.

Now look back at the supine plain film (see Fig. 2–72) and observe that the diagnosis of free peritoneal air can be very strongly suspected from this film alone. The dark vertical shadow far to the left is much too dark to be flank stripe and does not have the appearance of contained air at all.

Mr. Handsaw was taken to surgery, where he was found to have a perforated diverticular abscess.

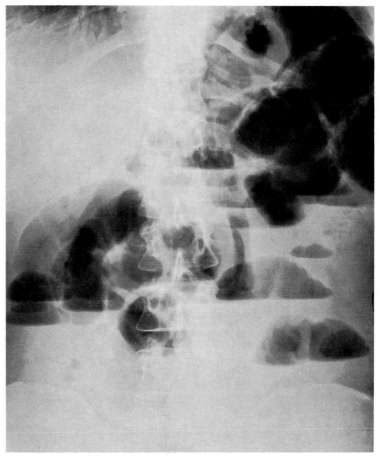

Figure 2–73   Mr. Handsaw, erect film, diaphragm not included.

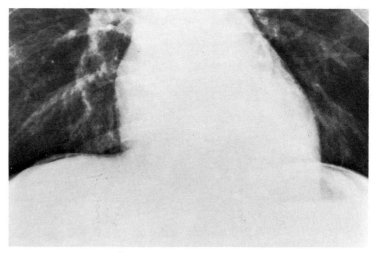

Figure 2–74   Mr. Handsaw, standing, film centered at diaphragm.

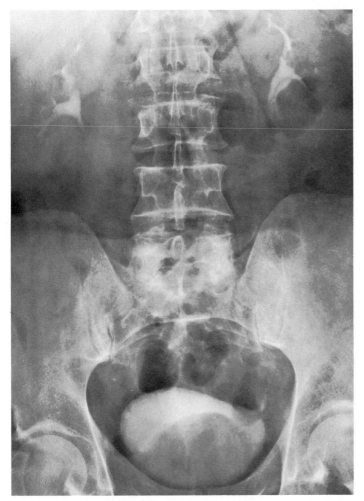

Figure 2–75 Aubrey Mandrake

Aubrey Mandrake, 69, magician, is seen in urology clinic because of grossly bloody urine for four days.

Roland Warlock, 45, mystery story writer, consults his doctor after being knocked down in the street by hoodlums who took his wallet. Returning home, he could discover no bruises or tenderness but observed that his urine was bright red.

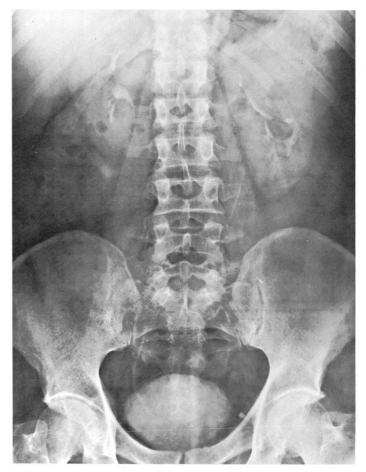

Figure 2–76 Roland Warlock

Harold Wolfbane, 51, exterminator, is referred from his place of employment because, after an unusually long day at work, he noticed that his urine was red. He is not particularly alarmed since other members of his family have been known to have the same symptom from time to time. They are all in clerical work and not exposed to toxins of any kind.

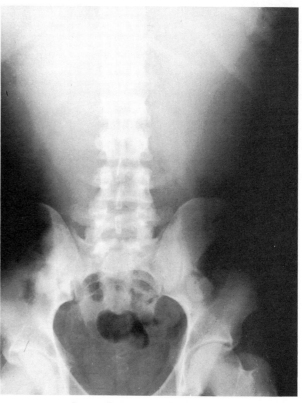

Figure 2–77 Harold Wolfbane

Answers

Mr. Mandrake's excretory urogram shows that both kidneys are normal in size and shape, and the calices appear nondilated, undistorted, and normally distributed within the kidney parenchyma. The ureters are not visible because of normal peristaltic activity, but the bladder shows a smooth defect arising from its floor typical of benign prostatic hypertrophy, one of the common causes of hematuria in elderly men. (The prostatic shadow here is too wide and too confined to the lower half of the bladder to be an overlying rectal bubble.)

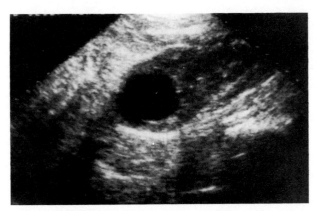

Figure 2–78 Warlock, renal ultrasound.

Mr. Warlock's presenting story suggests that his hematuria may be traumatic in origin, not at all an uncommon occurrence. However, the excretory urogram shows a large mass in the upper pole of the left kidney. The upper part of the collecting system is draped around this mass and distorted by it in a manner much more consistent with a longstanding intrarenal mass than with an acute hematoma. Moreover, the sharp take-off of the lower margin of this mass from the lateral margin of the kidney would be most unusual in acute injury to a previously normal kidney.

The differential diagnosis here is between solitary renal cyst and renal tumor, either of which may cause hematuria. Ultrasound examination showed a solitary, spherical, sonolucent mass consistent with a benign renal cyst (Fig. 2–78).

Mr. Wolfbane has very large kidney shadows on the supine abdominal film. His diagnosis was established as polycystic kidney disease on abdominal CT (Fig. 2–79). A sister and an aunt were also found to have polycystic kidneys.

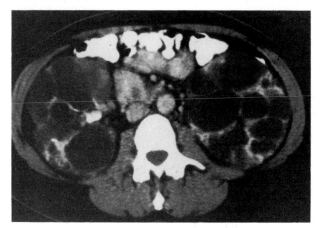

Figure 2–79 Wolfbane, abdominal CT.

Answers

Mr. Major has three different causes for pain and hematuria, all evident from the roentgen findings on a single abdominal plain film (Fig. 2–86). He has diffuse and patchy increased density of the bony pelvis, lumbar vertebrae, and upper femora. The increased thickness of bone seen in Paget's disease is not seen here, and the bone changes are most probably due to metastases from carcinoma of the prostate. There is also a large laminated bladder calculus, and, just above the symphysis pubis, a cluster of smaller calculi characteristic of the appearance of prostatic stones.

Dorothy Lewis's supine abdominal film shows a small calcification in the right kidney area (Fig. 2–87). Bowel gas is apparent in the stomach and colonic areas. Look very carefully at the left upper abdomen. Is the air in the left upper abdomen all in the colon or stomach? Figure 2–89A is the same abdominal film with arrows pointing out air in the left renal collecting system, around the left kidney, and even in the left proximal ureter.

This patient had a severe infection with a gas-producing organism *(Escherichia coli)*, causing the plain film findings. CT confirmed an extensive renal and perirenal abscess (Fig. 2–89B). The right-sided calcification is a calculus, nonobstructing. Because of the advanced destruction of the left kidney, nephrectomy was performed. Had she presented earlier with an intrarenal abscess, percutaneous drainage may have been curative. A few weeks later she was back to playing piano.

Mr. Lovelace's plain film (Fig. 2–88) was, of course, the preliminary one from an excretory urogram study and is normal except that the outline of the right kidney is much more clearly seen than the left and the kidney seems slightly larger in both length and thickness. The excretory study at 30 minutes (Fig. 2–90) shows why. This is the prolonged nephrogram seen in acute ureteral obstruction. Although no ureteral calculus can be seen, the diagnosis is indisputable and appropriate treatment must be planned. A *radiolucent* stone was passed spontaneously a few days later.

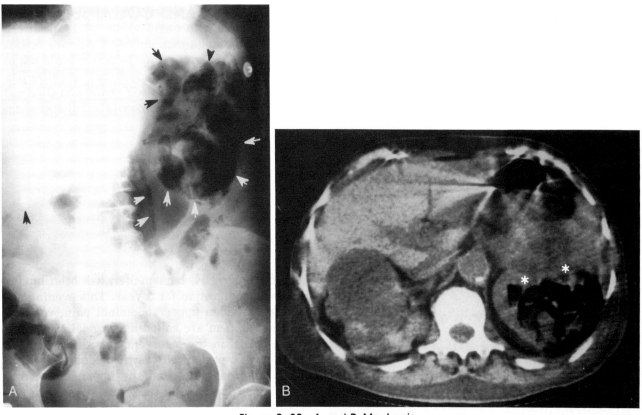

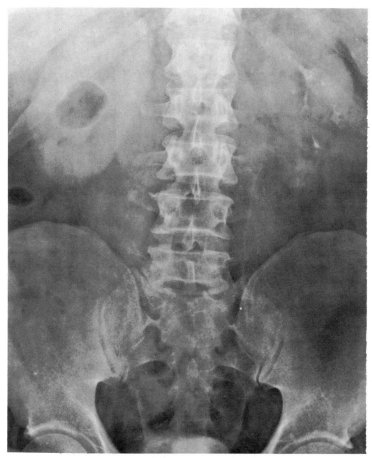

Figure 2–89 **A** and **B**, Mrs. Lewis

Figure 2–90 Mr. Lovelace, 30-minute urogram.

Answers

Mr. Mallone had a barium enema that shows abnormalities in the proximal transverse and sigmoid colon. According to the fluoroscopist, the transverse colonic area was in spasm. The sigmoid lesion is an irregular narrowing of the bowel lumen that persisted during fluoroscopic examination. It has the appearance of an adenocarcinoma, which it proved to be at surgery (Fig. 2–99; see also Fig. 2–102, with arrows).

Mr. Whipfelder's GI series (Fig. 2–100) shows the same lesser-curvature ulcer crater that was visible on his plain film. The fluoroscopist reports that it projects beyond the lumen of the stomach and that spot films show radiation of mucosal folds to the crater indicating a strong probability that it is benign. With medical treatment his symptoms abated within several days, and on repeat upper GI in 6 weeks the ulcer had resolved.

Miss Antoine's barium study is seen in Figure 2–101, three films of the duodenum. Have a go at them unaided.

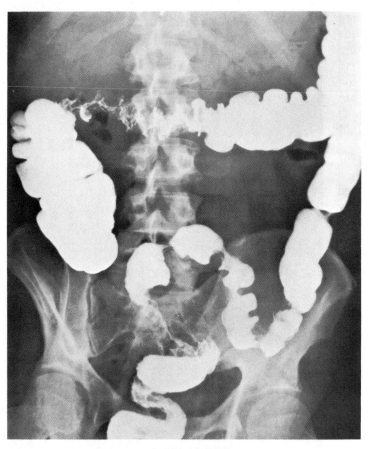

Figure 2–99 Mr. Mallone

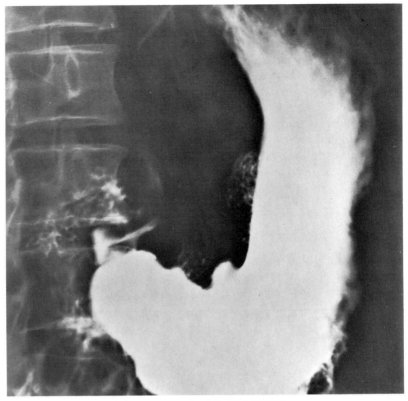

Figure 2–100 Mr. Whipfelder

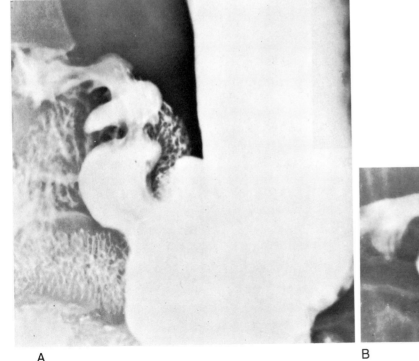

A

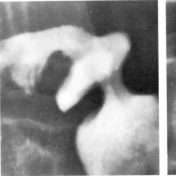

B

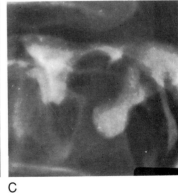

C

Figure 2–101 A to C, Miss Antoine.

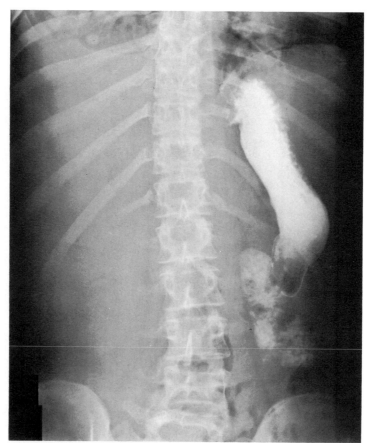

Figure 2–111

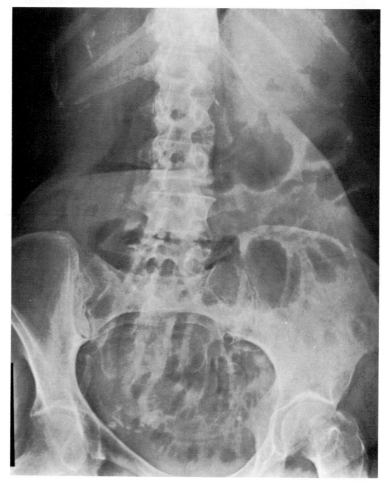

Figure 2–112

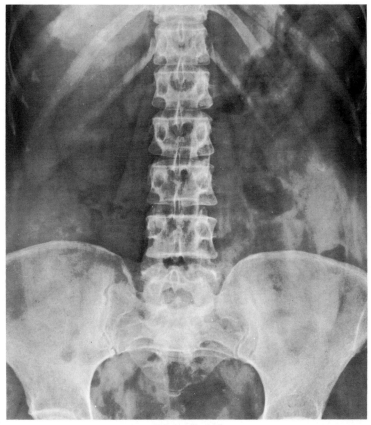

Figure 2–113

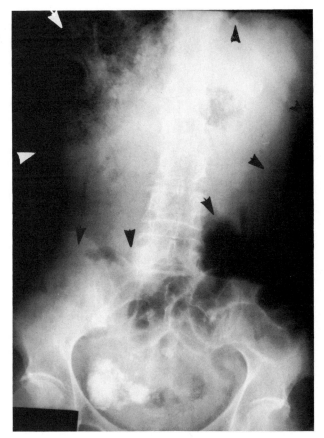

Figure 2–114

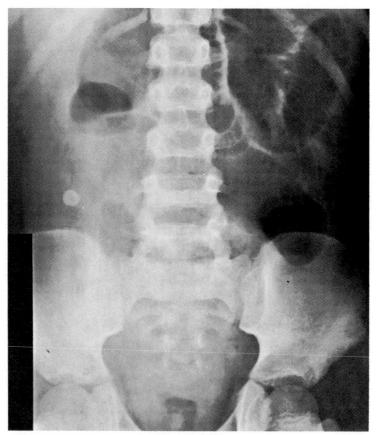

Figure 2–115

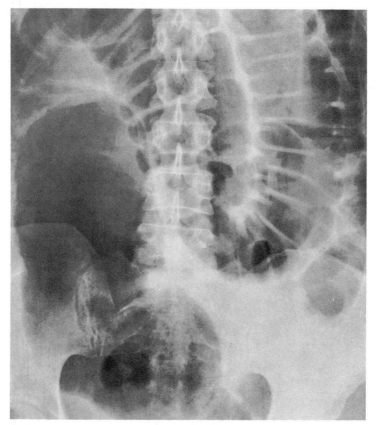

Figure 2–116

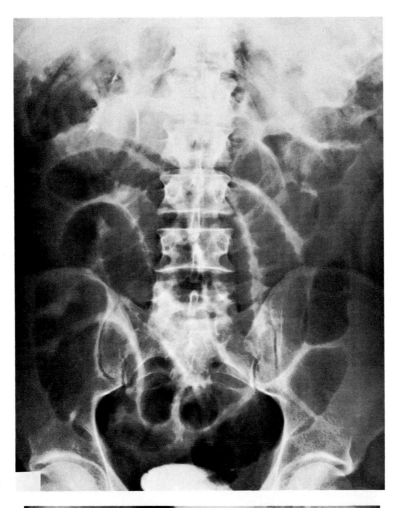

Figure 2–117

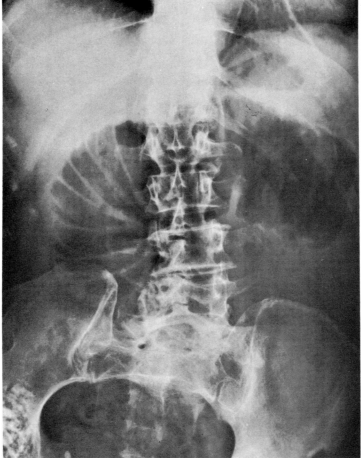

Figure 2–118

Answers

FIGURE 2–104

Figure 2–104 is a supine abdominal film on a young man who developed abdominal pain while in police custody. Note the opaque foreign body in the left lower quadrant. Several hours later the patient passed a crack vial in his bowel movement.

FIGURE 2–105

This abdominal plain film of a woman of 60 shows three greatly distended loops of jejunum in the midabdomen. There are also a few bubbles and a generalized grayness of the lower abdomen suggesting there may be other loops of small bowel filled with fluid. There is no air in the colon and no rectal bubble. The roentgen findings are those of advanced small bowel obstruction with complete clearing of the colon. Prompt surgical exploration is indicated. (At laparotomy, an adhesive band was found across a mid-ileal loop; lysis of the band relieved the obstruction at once. The patient made an excellent recovery.)

FIGURE 2–106

This is a supine abdominal film of a 67-year-old woman with a long history of mitral valvular heart disease who presented with severe acute abdominal pain and bloody diarrhea. The abdominal film is quite unremarkable. Fecaloid material is apparent in the rectum and cecum. Because of signs of peritonitis she had surgery. At surgery she was found to have a gangrenous cecum. Most of the time, fecaloid material will be just that, but a history of severe abdominal pain with accompanying bloody diarrhea and a history of heart disease should alert you to the possible diagnosis of ischemic bowel disease with necrosis. Ischemic bowel may mimic fecal material.

FIGURE 2–107

This abdominal plain film shows distended large and small bowel. The patient was postoperative one day after an oöphorectomy. Peristalsis was intermittent and decreased. A clinical diagnosis of adynamic ileus was being entertained, but the patient was sent to the x-ray department during the evening because of repeated complaints of abdominal pain and obvious distension. The films were felt to be reassuring, a confirmation of the impression of ileus, and the patient was managed conservatively. The next morning peristalsis was re-established and the patient made a good recovery.

FIGURE 2–108

On this plain film the liver and spleen both appear to be enlarged and the stomach air shadow is displaced downward between them. The small bowel contains more air than normal but is not distended. The patient had myelogenous leukemia.

FIGURE 2–109

This plain film shows distended small bowel loops in midabdomen, dilated cecum and ascending and transverse colon, but no air in descending colon or sigmoid and none in the rectum. The roentgen findings suggest large bowel obstruction at the splenic flexure and clearing below that point consistent with the clinical picture of gradually increasing constipation and distension. Barium enema showed an annular carcinoma just below the splenic flexure.

FIGURE 2–110

The plain film on this patient shows the stomach air shadow displaced to the left, metallic stay sutures in the RUQ, and air in small bowel, cecum, and transverse colon. There are also branching dark streaks over both right and left lobes of the liver suggesting air in the biliary tree. Without any clinical data it is impossible to say from this film whether the patient has had recent or remote gallbladder surgery. Either a surgical anastomosis or a spontaneous fistula can fill the biliary tree with air. In point of fact, surgery had been several months before and the patient had been readmitted to the hospital for terminal care because of widespread metastases from a melanosarcoma of the eye. At postmortem, the liver was enlarged and displaced the stomach far to the left.

FIGURE 2–111

This GI series is from a patient with a massive liver filled with metastases from an adrenal carcinoma. Note that the stomach is displaced far to the left. The bases of the lungs also show disseminated densities suggesting metastases.

FIGURE 2–112

This abdominal plain film shows greatly distended central loops of bowel, probably jejunum, and no air in the large bowel. Note that the mucosal markings are thickened and the loops separated, a finding that should often raise the question of ischemic bowel disease. At exploration, this 68-year-old woman had a strangulated femoral hernia, which had not been suspected clinically. The entire small bowel was gangrenous and the peritoneum contained three liters of bloody fluid. The patient died on the operating table.

FIGURE 2–113

This is a normal abdomen. The liver tip, right kidney, psoas shadows, and flank stripes are all normal. A scattering of air in stomach and bowel appears normal. No unusual masses or calcifications are seen.

FIGURE 2–114

This 73-year-old woman was brought to the emergency room by her elderly brother, who found her unconscious on the kitchen floor. On physical examination, her pulse was 120, blood pressure was 50/0, her temperature was 102° F. She had a distended abdomen with massive hepatomegaly, crepitance, and rebound tenderness. Her hemoglobin (Hb) was 6, Hct 18, WBC 21,000.

The supine abdominal film demonstrates air and fecaloid material in the RUQ, linear lucent lines, which represent air in intrahepatic veins, and a massively enlarged liver (arrows point to the liver edge). A calcified fibroid is in the pelvis. The patient was believed to have a liver abscess in a massively enlarged liver. Before any emergency diagnosis or treatment could be instituted, she died. At autopsy, she was found to have a massively enlarged liver filled with necrotic material caused by a carcinoma of the hepatic flexure that had infiltrated into the liver and necrosed because of a lack of adequate blood supply. Clostridia were also cultured from the necrotic liver.

FIGURE 2–115

This plain film from a child (as suggested by unfused pelvic epiphyses) has a round calcific shadow on the right and distended loops of small bowel. All bowel appears to be displaced out of the RLQ. At operation, a gangrenous appendix was found lying in a large periappendiceal abscess, which also contained a calcified fecalith.

FIGURE 2–116

This plain film shows a greatly distended large bowel from the cecum down to the distal descending colon, where there is an abrupt termination of the air shadow. Barium enema showed the presence of an annular carcinoma at this point.

FIGURE 2–117

This excretory urogram shows normal nondilated draining structures on the right and opaque material filling the bladder. No draining structures can be distinguished for the left kidney. There is a marked degree of reflex ileus present. With the clinical story of sudden flank pain and colic on the left, the findings suggest acute ureteral obstruction, and Figure 2–119 shows the late dense nephrogram that clinches that diagnosis. A very small calculus was passed the next day.

FIGURE 2–118

Plain film shows a single, greatly distended loop jejunum. There is also marked pelvic distortion and very old right hip disease. Figure 2–120 shows a large scrotal hernia also containing distended small bowel. At surgery the bowel was found to be dark and discolored but revived after the hernia was reduced. The patient made an excellent recovery.

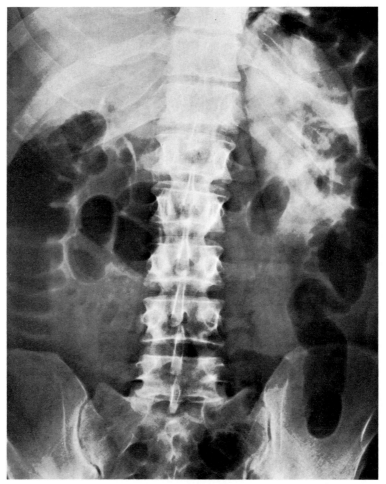

Figure 2–119

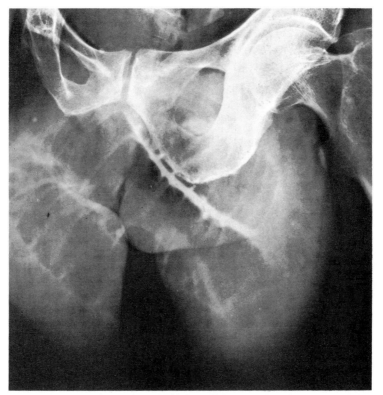

Figure 2–120

3 | Bone

Introduction

It may now be difficult for you to recall your bewilderment when first confronted with radiographs of the chest and abdomen. The apparently endless variety of shape, size, density, and lucency has by this time yielded to systematic analysis, sharpened powers of observation, and, surely, increased knowledge of anatomy and physiology. Doubts may return when you face the fact that, though an individual has but one chest and one abdomen, he or she has 206 bones (more or less), all of them different in size, shape, and function. Generations of unfortunate medical students have spent many hours committing to memory all the protuberances, ridges, notches, and processes of bone.

Let us celebrate together the declining popularity of such activity and proceed to a consideration of what bones really are—a uniform organ system with intricate structural and functional connections with all other organ systems in the body.

In correlating roentgen changes in bone with pathology, you will be happy to know that what you see in radiographs of bones indicates much more definitely what the histopathologic change is likely to be than in the chest and abdomen. For example, you will remember that there were any number of reasons why the right lower lobe might collapse or consolidate. Contrast with this the fact that the radiographic changes in the hands in such diverse conditions as acromegaly, hyperparathyroidism, and thalassemia major are so characteristic that one may immediately make those diagnoses. In most cases this can be done without benefit of historical record, physical examination, or laboratory findings. In fact, the radiographic changes in a good many

conditions are so specific that the pathologist, limited to a single bone biopsy specimen, consults the radiologist about his impression of the entire lesion before offering a final analysis of the tissue.

Because bone carries its own built-in contrast substance—calcium—changes in density and texture, once they occur, are readily visible even to the untrained eye.

You will first encounter, in Part A, a series of pagespreads having problems, usually related to each other, along with some clinical data. Each of these will be followed by answer pagespreads supplying comparable normals.

Part B will introduce you to an additional technique for learning, which we like to call "comparison shopping." This is an extension of the procedure in Part A, but instead of comparing a single normal with a single abnormal film, here we will offer you a number of radiographs of the same region, so that you can observe the tremendous range of roentgen changes that may occur. From this type of comparison you can appreciate rapid changes that even a radiologist might not see during the course of many months of routine daily work.

Part C will be a somewhat more didactic consideration of the fascinating process of bone growth and maintenance. A group of illustrative disease conditions will follow, in which bone growth is greatly altered. Many of the important metabolic conditions affecting bone will be presented in this section.

With all the foregoing under your belt, you will be ready for Part D, a series of mixed problems arranged in no particular sequence, as they might be encountered in the course of your daily practice.

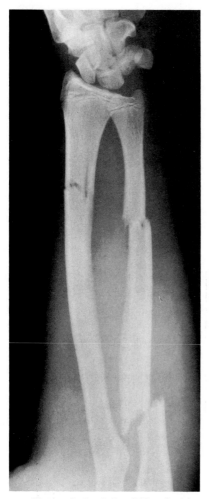

Figure 3–1 John O'Grady

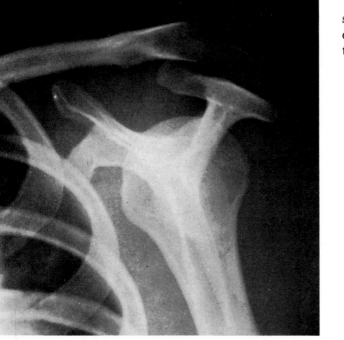

Figure 3–2 Henry Kowalski

Part A

Introductory Problems

These first four patients were a few of 30 victims of a 20-car pileup occurring on the Harbor Freeway (substitute any other) at rush hour during the worst rain storm of the year. Many are complaining of pain, and after physical examination you have requested the appropriate x-ray examinations.

John O'Grady is still not fully conscious as a result of a head injury, but you note that his left forearm is very swollen and shows ecchymoses. Gentle palpation is very painful.

Henry Kowalski walks in with his left arm in a sling. He informs you that the pain is in the shoulder. You note a tender, very localized swelling at the lateral end of the clavicle.

Alex Kowalski, his brother, did not get hurt, but thinks that while he is there, you might take a look at his right hand.

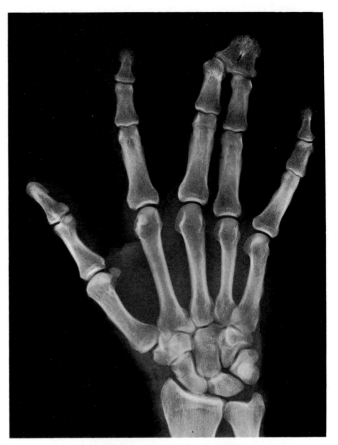

Figure 3–3 Alex Kowalski

Joanna Johnstone walks in, limping. She has pain in her knee but is more concerned about her bruised nose. You request x-rays of both the nose and her knee. Films of the nose prove to be normal. Here is the one of the lower extremity. What do you think of it?

(Look at all four of these problem cases and try to decide what is wrong before turning to the answer pagespread.)

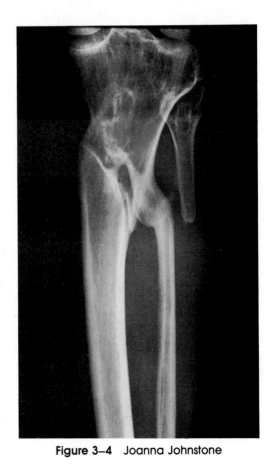

Figure 3–4 Joanna Johnstone

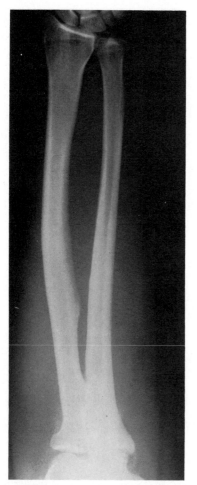

Figure 3–5 Normal forearm.

Answers

The most common and impressive change in bone one can encounter is, without doubt, the fracture. *Mr. O'Grady* has fractures of both bones of the forearm. Fractures, as traumatic interruptions in the continuity of bone, have a wide range of x-ray appearance, some of which you will encounter later in the series of exercises. Is Figure 3–5 Mr. O'Grady's other forearm? (Answer in box below.)

No, Figure 3–5 is not Mr. O'Grady's other forearm. The patient in Figure 3–5 is much older than Mr. O'Grady because he has closed epiphyses. Note in Mr. O'Grady's film (Fig. 3–1) the difference between the abrupt interruption in continuity of the fracture and the white-margined, unfused, epiphyseal growth plates of the distal radius and ulna. This will be obvious if you tip the page so that you can view Figures 3–1 and 3–5 side by side.

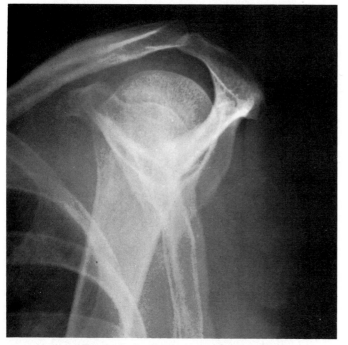

Figure 3–6 Normal shoulder.

Figure 3–6 is *Henry Kowalski's* uninjured shoulder (photographically reversed) for comparison. Figure 3–2 shows no fracture—no interruption of bone. But there *is* an abnormality of positional relationship of one bone to another—an acromioclavicular dislocation.

(To make direct comparison of one film with another, place the margin of page 176 in the center of page 174. You may use this method throughout the book.)

Alex Kowalski's other hand was normal. It was obvious from your clinical examination that he had a congenital fusion of the soft tissues of his third and fourth digits. The radiograph adds the information that the bones are also fused. (Compare Alex's hand with Figure 3–15 in which the tips of the third and fourth fingers were intentionally overlapped.)

We have not felt it necessary to illustrate a normal hand for you here. An abnormality involving only one digit can be compared with other digits in the same hand. Remember this principle when examining films of vertebrae or ribs.

Mrs. Johnstone had been hit by a car 10 years ago and has had pain in her knee (in damp weather) ever since. Figure 3–7 is a normal leg. There had been a large confluent hematoma surrounding the fractures of the tibia and fibula at the time of the original injury. As we shall see in other fractures, the hematoma provides a base for the deposition of bone (callus) for the purpose of healing. The process has resulted here in a smooth fusion of the fibula to the tibia. Note that the original fracture line in the tibia is still visible, though bridged by bone.

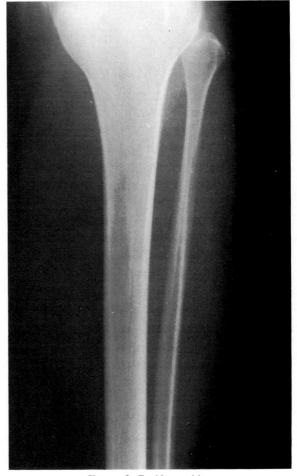

Figure 3–7 Normal leg.

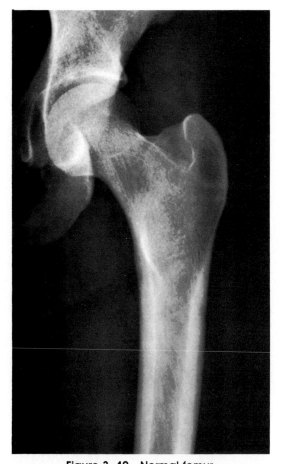

Figure 3–12 Normal femur.

Answers

When compared with the normal femur in Figure 3–12, *Mr. Widner's* femur is notably bowed. There is also a relative increase in roentgen density of the bone. This is most obvious in the shaft (or diaphysis) where apparent overgrowth of rather featureless compact bone has begun to encroach on the dark shadow of the medullary cavity. Overgrowth is also centrifugal, resulting in a net increase in diameter of the shaft from new subperiosteal bone formation. In the head and neck of the femur, the fine trabeculae of the normal bone (Fig. 3–12) are in marked contrast to the irregularly arranged, coarse trabeculae of the diseased bone. Because the abnormal bone of Paget's disease (which *Mr. Widner* has) is of poor structural strength, a gradual lateral bowing of the femur has resulted. You will most often recognize Paget's disease in its chronic healing phase when the bone is thickened and the trabecular pattern distorted. Lucent lines partway across the bone, sometimes seen in Paget's disease, are known as "pseudofractures." Look back at the detail view in Figure 3–8: Mr. Widner has a pseudofracture in the lateral cortex.

Jerry Stoner, who is four years old, shows symmetrical, anterior bowing of both tibias (healed rickets). Two years ago he was suffering from active rickets. Because of severe dietary vitamin D deficiency he was unable to absorb enough calcium from his intestine to adequately mineralize his bones, hence the bowing. Note how the thickness of the posterior cortex is being correctively increased,

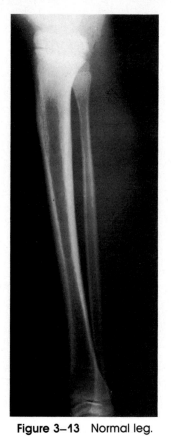

Figure 3–13 Normal leg.

eventually to offset the bowing. This is called re-modeling.

Mr. Boos' fibula is congenitally absent except for the small, misshapen remnant of bone at the distal end of the extremity. Though the fibula is a non-weight-bearing bone, it does provide a locus of attachment for many muscle groups. The final adult shape of any bone is the result of many forces, not the least of which is muscular pull. In the absence of the fibula, there has been a marked rearrange-ment of muscular tension vectors, resulting in an unusually shaped tibia and what appears to be a grossly unstable knee joint.

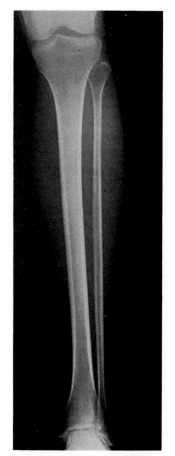

Figure 3–14 Normal leg.

Acquired absence of bone is much more common. *Mr. Dreiser* had fractured the navicular bone of his wrist. Because of peculiarities in the blood supply to that bone, his fracture failed to heal, resulting in a painful wrist. Removal of the dead bone is often the only satisfactory treatment. The film of the wrist (Fig. 3–11) was made immediately following re-moval of a heavily autographed plaster cast, which had been in place for six weeks. Comparison with the normal wrist in Figure 3–15 makes more easily visible the marked "demineralization" of the distal radius, ulna, and remaining carpal bones. This is *bone loss* as a result of absent muscular pull, or, as commonly termed, *atrophy of disuse.* "Demineraliza-tion" is a much abused term in common use and it should be avoided. It is misleading because it im-plies loss of mineral in still existing bone rather than a net decrease in bone mass—the actual state of affairs. Note the superimposition of greater on lesser multangular and of pisiform on triquetrum.

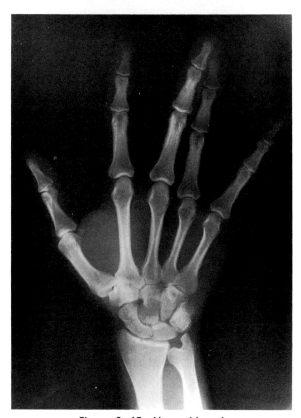

Figure 3–15 Normal hand.

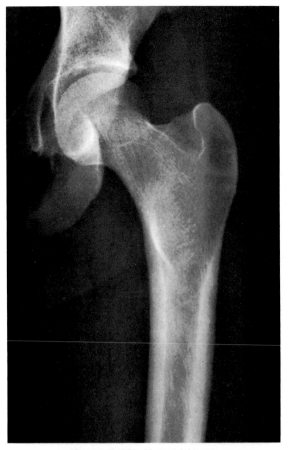

Figure 3–28 Normal femur.

Answers

Although their histories differ, *Mr. Silver's* stump, *Ms. McGillicuddy's* right leg, and *Mrs. Plunkett's* femur are osteoporotic because of disuse. These three patients illustrate that bone put to rest for any reason whatsoever will soon show a net loss of matrix along with its minerals.

As is clearly seen in *Mr. Silver's* stump, the loss of bone is not uniform throughout. The cortex of the femoral shaft is thin, and its delimitation from spongiosa is less sharp. There is a patchy, irregular loss of roentgen density in both cortex and spongy bone, where whole chunks of matrix and mineral have been resorbed. On histologic examination, the bone that is left would appear quite normal. The marked shortening and broadening of the femoral neck in Figure 3–24 are undoubtedly due to an old, healed fracture.

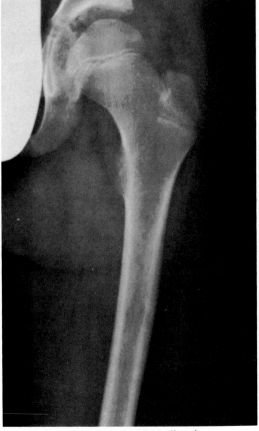

Figure 3–29 Hilda's other leg.

Ms. McGillicuddy's polio has markedly reduced the functioning muscle mass in her entire right lower extremity. In the absence of muscle pull, there is not only osteoporosis but also underdevelopment. For example, compare directly the capital femoral epiphysis and greater trochanter on the normal left side (Fig. 3–29).

Mrs. Plunkett's fracture shows exuberant callus formation. Again, the typical changes of osteoporosis are present in the bone on either side of the fracture itself.

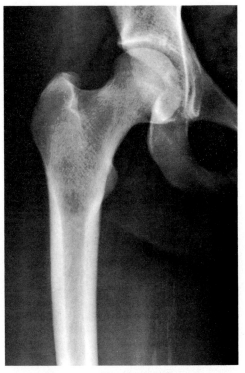

Figure 3–30 Normal femur.

Mr. Hong's problem is entirely different. He has not been injured; he has no loss of neuromuscular power; he leads an active life; yet he is losing bone. Though we have warned you against accepting any fixed combination of roentgen findings as being typical of any particular disease, here you may throw caution to the winds and exclaim, "Hyperparathyroidism!"—for these roentgen findings are truly pathognomonic. In addition to cortical thinning, coarsening, and reduction in the number of trabeculae in the spongiosa, there is also a peculiar resorption of the superficial layers of cortex in the phalanges (Fig. 3–31, arrows).

The pattern of resorption results in a fine irregularity of the bony outline often described as "lacy." (Figure 3–31 gives you a detail from Figure 3–27, with a normal for direct comparison.)

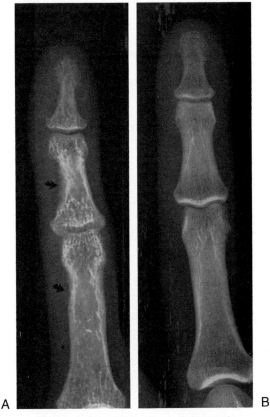

A   B

Figure 3–31 A, Mr. Hong. B, Normal.

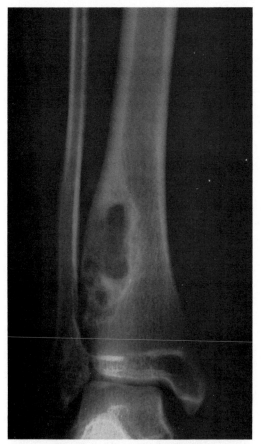

Figure 3–32 Jennifer Potter

FOUR PATIENTS WITH SOLITARY LESIONS

Jennifer Potter is a 17 year old who fell down the school steps and sprained her ankle. She had no complaints prior to the injury.

Ria Giovanetti, 57, is complaining of pain in her forearm that she cannot relate to any injury. She tells you that her left kidney had been removed five years ago because of a "tumor."

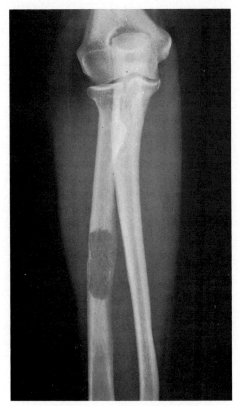

Figure 3–33 Ria Giovanetti

Henry Darnley is a 35-year-old plumber who, for eight years, has had a gradually increasing dull aching pain in his left knee that he attributes to long kneeling under kitchen sinks. He is limping slightly as he walks into your office.

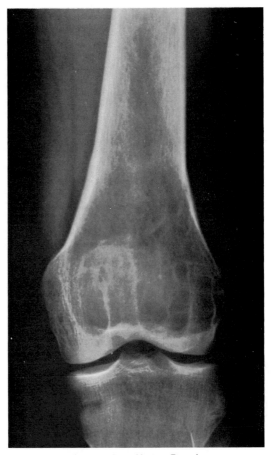

Figure 3–34   Henry Darnley

Robert Dudley, 26, a heroin addict, has also had increasing pain in his left knee. He has ignored it even though it has become so severe that his mobility is limited. He appears in the emergency room after having been struck by a slowly moving car. You note tenderness over the patella and a large, hard, slightly tender mass above the knee.

All these patients suffer from tumors of bone. Can you tell:

1. Which are benign and which malignant?
2. In which there has been expansion of cortex?
3. In which there has been periosteal response?
4. In which there is invasion into surrounding soft tissues? What is wrong with the proximal tibia in Figure 3–35?

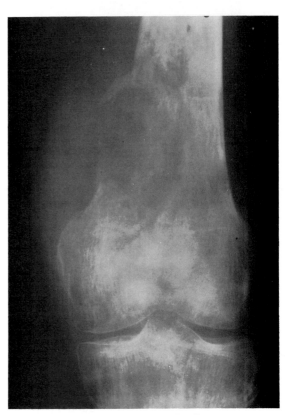

Figure 3–35   Bob Dudley

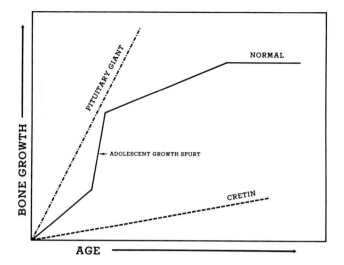

Figure 3–73 Curves of normal and abnormal bone growth.

Until recently, knowledge about how bones grow has been limited by the methods of investigation available—anatomic sections and a few notable animal studies. (See historical note on the next page.) Roentgen's discovery was a tremendous stimulus to investigation, because now one could study the appearance of any bone as a continuing progression. Though this method provides only gross anatomic facts, it has given rise to much information of a practical clinical nature. For instance, it is now an accepted clinical tool to obtain serial roentgenograms of a specific part of the anatomy, match them against standard normals, and plot them as points on a curve—an index to the *rate* of skeletal growth and maturation.

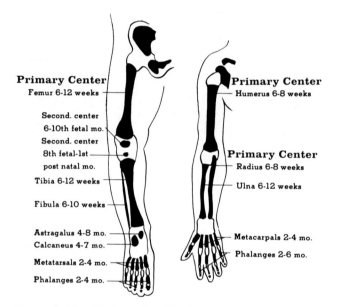

Figure 3–74 Centers of ossification normally present at birth and their appearance times during fetal life (after Caffey).

An account of the events in bone maturation starts at the *fetal* age of six weeks, when the initial changes leading to ossification commence in the cartilaginous anlage for the tibia.

These foci are known as *primary centers of ossification.* Figure 3–74 will give you some idea of the order of appearance of these centers. Usually, just before birth, the first of the *secondary centers of ossification* appears on both sides of the knee—the distal femur and the proximal tibia. Of course, from this point on, growth in length of bones occurs at the *growth plate* (or physis)—the junction between primary and secondary centers of ossification.

John Belchier's Dinner Guest

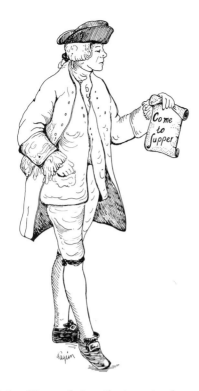

Imagine yourself transported backward in time to 1736. You have been invited to dine (at three in the afternoon) with Mr. John Belchier, an English surgeon. It is the England of George I, who speaks only German; the England of Hogarth and Handel and Dr. Johnson. The microscope has made it possible to see minute organisms, but man still believes in their spontaneous generation! Half of all the children in London die before their fifth year, and the average life expectancy is only 22 years. Most English physicians still reject inoculation for smallpox, 20 years after its introduction from Turkey. Of course, your host is not even a physician: surgeons have not yet been elevated from the society of barbers, and Voltaire has said that of 100 doctors, 98 are charlatans.

Not being able to afford a sedan chair, you go on foot, dressed in a frock coat and knee breeches, buckled shoes, and a three-cornered hat, your hair shoulder length, tied back with a neat bow at the nape of your neck. The company of six men are friends of Mr. Belchier, who has requested that a suckling pig be brought up from his farm in the country and roasted for your delectation.

As he bids you be seated, the servant utters an exclamation at the sideboard where he is carving the pig onto pewter plates. He draws the attention of his master to the fact that the exposed bones are brilliant rose-colored, although the meat is well done and not pink itself. Belchier demands an explanation. The master of livestock from the farm is brought in. He explains that yesterday he carried the pig up to town and that some time ago this litter of pigs accidentally got into a bin containing dried madder, used to dye stockings red. He remembers the small pigs' snouts stained red when they were discovered. This happened, he says, about a fortnight ago.

Mr. Belchier is sure that in some curious way the stain has "taken" in the bones and not elsewhere and announces that he will conduct some "experiments" at the farm. It is an era when experiments are performed, even by laymen. You are interested, but not really impressed, being concerned about more mundane matters. You have no idea that you have witnessed an accident that, within 20 years or so, in the hands of Duhamel in France and John Hunter here at home, will have afforded an explanation of just how bones grow.

Up to now men have believed that bone growth is "interstitial" in character; that is, new bone grows within and displaces existing bone. ("Interstitial" growth is typical of soft parenchymatous organs such as the liver.)

Eleven years ago Hales proved that bones grow in *length* at their ends. He drilled holes a measured distance apart in the midshaft of a young chicken's leg and found, several months later, that the holes were exactly the same distance apart. (Two hundred years hence, radiology will make this sort of measurement much easier—something else you do not even dream of as you trudge home.)

Soon John Hunter will repeat the madder-feeding experiments under controlled conditions in a whole litter of pigs, which he will kill serially, showing that long bones grow in *thickness* by adding new bone under the periosteum. It is this recently formed bone—accidentally stained—that you have just been privileged to "see" for the first time in history. Figure 3–75 shows you the cross sections of femurs from Hunter's litter of *serially sacrificed* pigs. You can deduce the conduct of the experiment and its precise implications if you know that the stippled areas were stained bright red. (Belchier and his dinner party are well-documented fact, not fiction.)

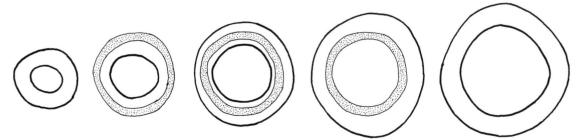

Figure 3–75   John Hunter's pigs; cross sections of femur.

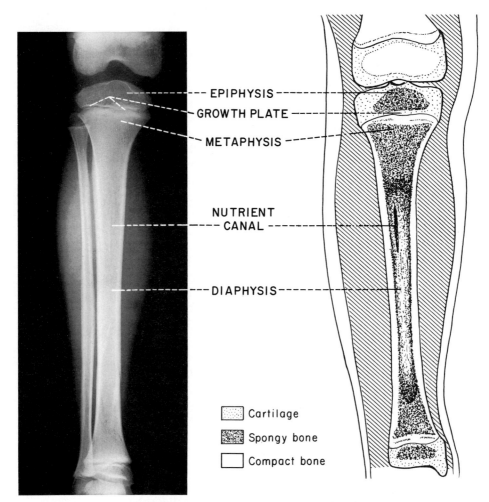

Figure 3–76 Parts of a growing bone (after Caffey).

Figure 3–76 shows a radiograph of a growing tibia. The accompanying line drawing will identify for you the parts to which we will refer during the discussion that follows.

A growing long bone has four anatomic subdivisions of concern in normal and abnormal bone growth. These subdivisions are functionally differentiated from one another. Each contributes in a different way to the form of the adult bone. As a corollary, then, diseases of growing bone are often identifiable because they affect a specific part. For example, in Velasquez' "Las Meninas" (Fig. 3–77), can you find a figure who has a disease that affects the proliferating cartilage of the growth plate?

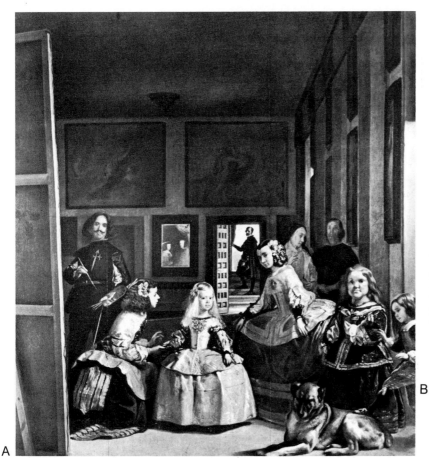

A

Figure 3–77 A, Velasquez' "Las Meninas" ("The Ladies-in-Waiting").

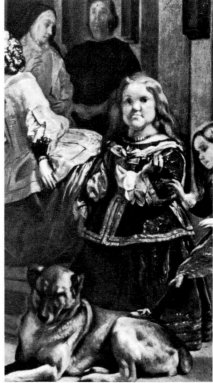

B

Figure 3–77 B, Detail (age 29 years).

Much sought after as servant and clown in the sixteenth-century courts of Europe, the adult achondroplastic dwarf was considered attractive and amusing because of his grotesque appearance. The proliferating cartilage at the ends of long bones is deficient in amount and abnormal in structure in achondroplasia. The result is a bone much shorter than normal, but because there is no disturbance of periosteal function, the diameter of the *shaft* is quite normal, the bones thus appearing too thick relative to their length. Figure 3–78 is the hand of an achondroplast, aged six. Compare with the series of normals at the beginning of this section.

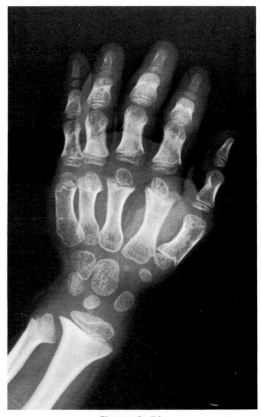

Figure 3–78

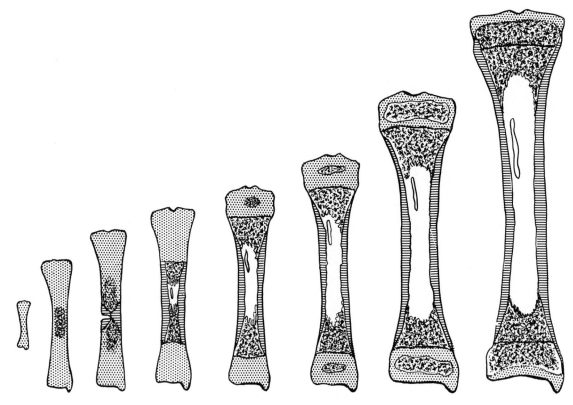

Figure 3–79 Growth of a bone (the tibia)—fetal anlage to maturity (after Caffey).

In all but a few bones of the human skeleton, ossification occurs when new bone matrix is applied, like plaster, against a supporting sponge of calcified cartilage. In the fetus the entire skeleton is cartilaginous until about the fetal age of six weeks. The first true bone formation occurs then, near the midshaft of long bones, such as the tibia (Fig. 3–79). The cartilage cells in the midshaft enlarge and proliferate. Blood vessels from the perichondrium invade the central shaft and mineral salts extracted from the blood are deposited in the new bone matrix. (The channel so created becomes the nutrient canal for the mature bone.) At the same time the perichondrium begins to deposit primitive bone around the circumference of the midshaft to form a narrow collar. The membrane can now be called the "periosteum."

At either end of the ossification center, cartilage continues to proliferate and new bone is applied to each succeeding layer of cartilage (increasing the length of the bone). As this process continues at the ends of the shaft, the medullary cavity is formed by resorption centrally.

The growth in diameter of the midshaft has already been diagrammed for you on page 213, in relation to the early vital staining experiments of Belchier and Hunter. The growth in the length of a bone is the result of a more complex process taking place at the growth plate.

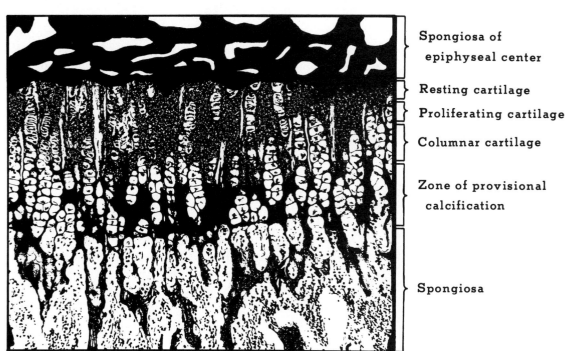

Figure 3–80 The growth plate seen microscopically.

Spongiosa of
epiphyseal center

Resting cartilage

Proliferating cartilage

Columnar cartilage

Zone of provisional
calcification

Spongiosa

Figure 3–80 is a diagrammatic representation of a microscopic section through a small portion of the growth plate. On the epiphyseal side of the growth plate is a layer of very young chondrocytes capable of self-replication. This layer of actively proliferating cells leaves in its wake layers of more mature cells, which rearrange themselves in queues separated by amorphous cartilaginous matrix. They then swell, vacuolate, and lyse, leaving an empty sponge of cartilage that has become provisionally calcified by mineral salts carried there by the invading blood vessels. *Remember, this is not bone; it is calcified cartilage.*

This layer of calcified cartilage is visible radiologically and referred to as the "zone of provisional calcification" (see Fig. 3–76). Only with deposition of a protein matrix by osteoblasts on these now-rigid girders of calcified cartilage is bone produced, mineralizing in its turn to form the trabecular struts of the metaphysis. Shaping and restructuring of these primary trabeculae results in a complex sponge of "cancellous bone."

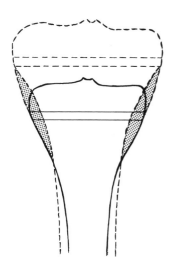

Figure 3–81 The enlarging metaphysis (after Weinmann and Sicher).

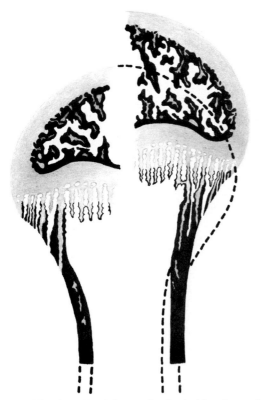

Figure 3–82 Growth of the metaphysis (structures shown in black represent true bone) (after Ham).

Thus, the metaphysis is seen on the radiograph as the flaring segment lying between shaft and the growth plate. It is composed almost entirely of trabecular bone. In the active weight-bearing organism, trabeculae arrange themselves most thickly along lines of maximum stress—a marvelous example of natural economy (Fig. 3–83).

At the periphery of the metaphysis at its junction with the growth plate, the production of *compact* bone by the active periosteum proceeds at such a pace that the metaphysis is constantly invested in a shell of compact bone. Thus, many of the peripherally placed marrow spaces are also filled in with compact bone. These processes, periosteal and endosteal together, result in formation of the tubular cortex of the whole bone, endowing it with great resistance to bending (compare the strength of a solid rod with that of a hollow pipe of the same diameter).

If periosteal compact bone formation proceeded unchecked, eventually a very thick cortex would be produced. However, in response to mechanical muscle pull and weight bearing, constant resorption and remodeling takes place. As shown in Figure 3–84, this process is most conspicuous at the metaphysis, resulting in a gradual, graceful constriction of the broad muscle-bearing metaphysis as it merges with the strong but slender, tubular, weight-bearing diaphysis.

The growth of the epiphysis or *secondary ossification center* of a long bone occurs by a process identical to that of the shaft. Here, instead of an advancing *disc* of cartilage at the growth plate (behind which ossification takes place), we have an expanding *sphere,* the surface of which is the site of cartilage-bone transformation, exactly the same as the transformation occurring at the growth plate.

This process continues until the epiphyseal cancellous bone abuts the mature metaphysis, at which time there is fusion and obliteration of the growth plate. At this point, further growth in length is no longer possible.

On the joint side of the epiphysis, endochondral production of bone stops short, leaving a shell of cartilage as a smooth, low-friction surface for the joint.

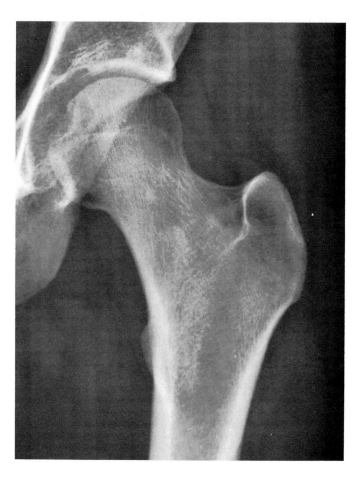

Figure 3–83 Normal arrangement of trabecular struts for weight bearing.

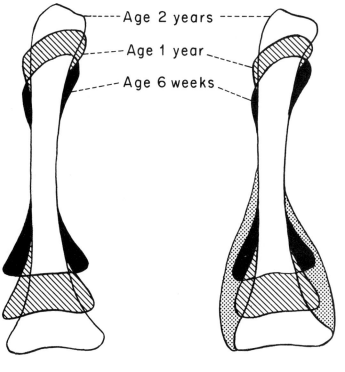

A. Modeled   B. Not modeled

Age 2 years
Age 1 year
Age 6 weeks

Figure 3–84 Diagrammatic representation of bone growth with **(A)** and without **(B)** modeling. The stippled bone in **B** is the bone that would have been removed by periosteal action if normal modeling had taken place (after Caffey).

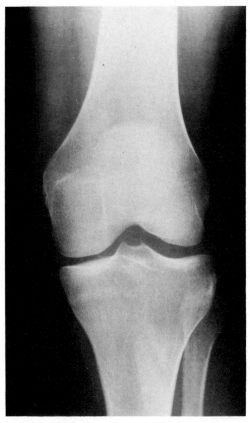

Figure 3–85 Distal femur.

Bones, then, lengthen, thicken, and model themselves as they grow and mature. No one of these processes can occur without the others, nor can these processes occur normally without the stimuli afforded by weight bearing, muscular pull, and endocrine secretion. Bone cannot form or be maintained without adequate supplies of calcium, phosphate, protein, and other nutrients.

Bone disease is therefore the result of a disturbance anywhere in this complex system. Some problems for you to analyze follow.

Modeling Problem

Figure 3–85 is a normal distal femur. Use it as a guide for deciding how the modeling process has been altered in both patients (Figs. 3–86 and 3–87). (We are not interested in having you attempt an exact diagnosis here!)

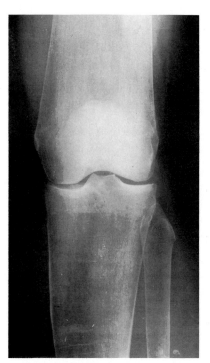

Figure 3–86

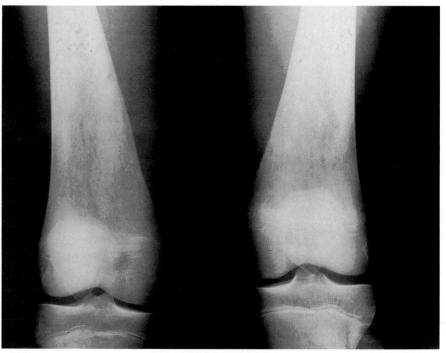

Figure 3–87

Answer

The two patients in Figures 3–86 and 3–87 had exactly the same modeling defect, but as the result of different mechanisms. Figure 3–86 is an example of an exceedingly rare congenital bone disease in which formation of the normal marrow cavity by removal of most newly formed spongy bone in the metaphysis fails to occur. The result is the accumulation of normal trabecular bone in increasing amounts, covered by only a thin shell of cortex. The cortex, of course, does not develop to its normal thickness because of the structural strength afforded by the overly abundant spongiosa. Microscopic examination of bone from patients with this condition shows nothing abnormal. The cause is still unknown. (The disease has an eponymic tag—Pyle's disease.)

In contrast to Pyle's disease, in which the abnormality is intrinsic to the skeleton, the bones of our second patient have modeling failure imposed upon them by a generalized metabolic disorder of the reticuloendothelial system (Gaucher's disease). The bone marrow of the metaphysis is an important part of that system. Microscopic sections of involved marrow show accumulation in huge numbers of large histiocytic cells with foamy cytoplasm, containing enormous quantities of a complex lipid material. In the growing individual with this disease, the capacity and stimuli for modeling (constriction of the shaft by periosteal action) are present, but they are overcome by the internal pressure of the ever-expanding mass of abnormal soft tissue cells. Spongy bone is also destroyed, resulting in weakness of the bone, very often leading to pathologic fracture.

Doubtless it seems to you that these two radiographs are very similar. In actual practice the differentiation of these two conditions would have to be made with the help of the clinical story. The patient with Pyle's disease is well; but the patient with Gaucher's disease has a metabolic fault with involvement of other organs, especially the liver and spleen. In patients with Gaucher's disease you might also find other skeletal manifestations, such as locally destructive expanding lesions, and aseptic necrosis, particularly of the femoral heads.

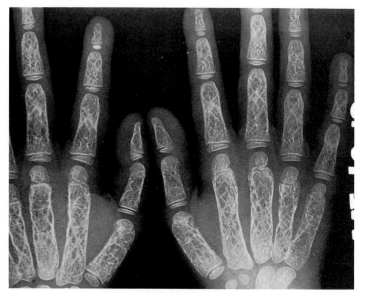

Figure 3-88   Rosa Di Napoli

Problems

The problems and answers on the next several pagespreads should be looked at while keeping in mind what you have already observed about bone growth and maturation. Decide which of the four parts (epiphysis, growth plate, metaphysis, diaphysis) of the growing bone is involved. Then decide whether there has been alteration of length, diameter, secondary center growth, or modeling. Once this is done, you will be well on the way to a diagnosis.

Rosa Di Napoli is an eight-year-old girl whose parents are becoming concerned that she has not grown as fast as other girls her age. She is pale and has a large head, and there is unusual prominence of the forehead. You find her hemoglobin 6 g per 100 ml and the peripheral blood smear markedly abnormal. Both parents are of Italian extraction and mildly anemic.

John Carrara is brought to you because of a severe nosebleed that required blood transfusion in the accident room. He is thin and very pale, and has an enlarged liver and spleen. Blood tests taken before transfusion show a reduction in numbers of all formed elements, including platelets.

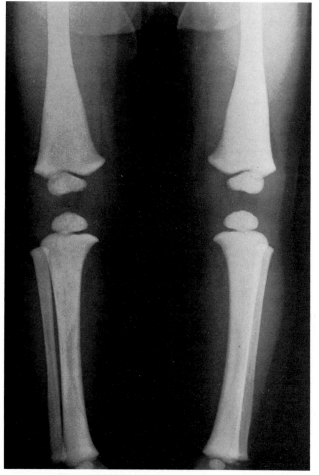

Figure 3-89   John Carrara, age 1.

Jimmy Hollis is ten years old and is well except for being slightly shorter than other boys his age. He injured his left hand playing baseball, and the films shown here were made.

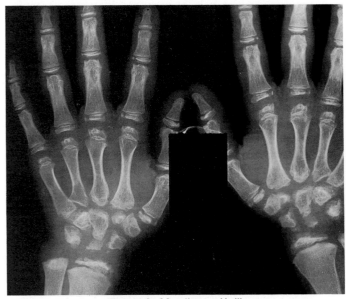

Figure 3–90   Jimmy Hollis

Janet Osgood is 17 years old. She is concerned because she walks with a limp. She has also noted that her left forearm is a little shorter than her right.

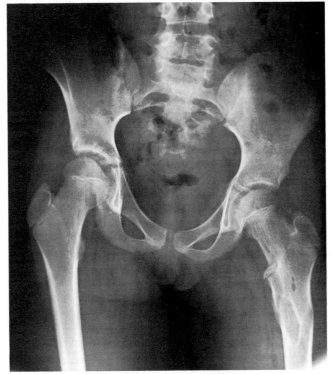

Figure 3–91   Janet Osgood

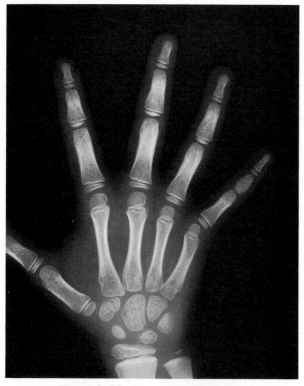

Figure 3-92 Normal child's hand.

Answers

Rosa Di Napoli's bones appear normal in length. The defect here is failure of modeling—a modeling failure very similar to what you have just seen in Gaucher's disease. The epiphyses seem normally developed. There is the striking additional finding of a markedly abnormal trabecular pattern, with coarsening and thickening of individual trabeculae as well as an overall reduction in their number. All these changes are the result of marrow hyperplasia in this patient with thalassemia major. Both parents were found to have thalassemia, but in a mild heterozygous form. No bone changes were seen in their films.

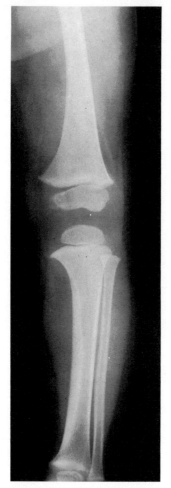

Figure 3-93 Normal child's leg.

Your first response, on seeing *John Carrara's* films, was to check the exposure factors with the technologist. He points out that the edge of the film is well blackened and that there is adequate penetration of the soft tissues.

After a second look it is apparent that there is no visible medullary cavity in the long bones, nor is there any visible trabeculation. Modeling of the distal femur is also abnormal. This patient has a disease known as osteopetrosis, or "marble bones." It is the result of failure of resorption of provisionally calcified cartilage and bone, so there is no space for marrow. The bone thus formed is of little structural value and is subject to spontaneous fracture. Production of formed blood elements is removed to the liver, spleen, and other reticuloendothelial organs. The modeling abnormality seen in the femur is also the result of delayed reconstruction of metaphyseal bone.

The changes in *Jimmy Hollis'* hand were typical of those seen in almost all his *epiphyseal* centers. Development of the shaft and metaphysis appears normal. The disease is known as multiple epiphyseal dysplasia and was found in other members of his family, all of whom were short in stature.

A normal film of the pelvis and proximal femur is not needed because *Janet Osgood's* right side is normal. The striking unilaterality of the changes provides a clue to the diagnosis of enchondromatosis, or Ollier's disease. In this condition, columns of proliferating cartilage originating at the growth plate fail to undergo normal endochondral bone formation and remain to disrupt the modeling and growth in length of the shaft.

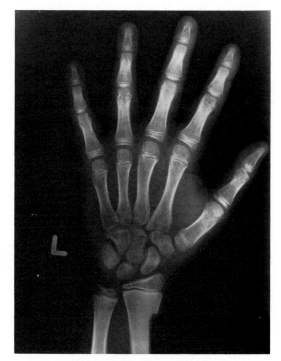

Figure 3–94 Normal hand.

Problems

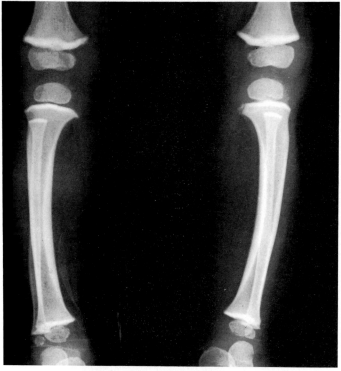

Figure 3–95 Patricia Plumb

Patricia Plumb, two years old, is brought to you by ambulance after a grand mal seizure. You examine her and find, upon funduscopic examination, evidence of increased intracranial pressure. Questioning the mother reveals that the child has the habit of eating bits of painted-over wall paper she pulls from the wall of their very old tenement apartment.

This film of *Billy Johnson's* forearm was made after he fell out of his jungle gym injuring his arm. You have requested films of other parts of his skeleton after seeing this one.

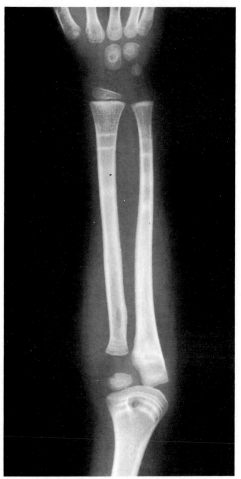

Figure 3–96 Billy Johnson, age 3.

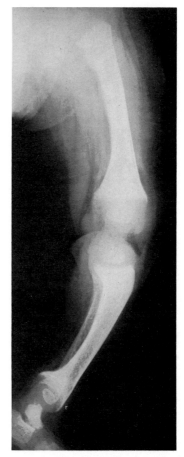

Figure 3–97   Ricky Stump, age 1.

The two children, *Ricky Stump* and *Mina See,* whose films you see on this page have been brought in to you by a child welfare worker who found both of them abandoned in a slum neighborhood. They appear chronically ill and are severely malnourished. *Ricky Stump* has lower extremities that are laterally bowed. You note tender swelling just beneath the skin of the thorax at the costochondral junctions. *Mina See's* skin is covered with large and small ecchymoses. You prove increased capillary fragility by a tourniquet test.

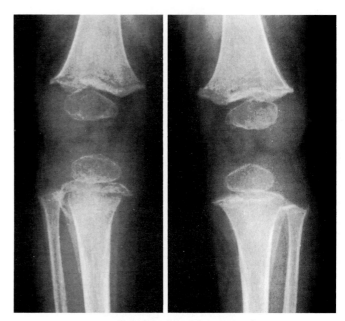

Figure 3–98   Mina See, age 1.

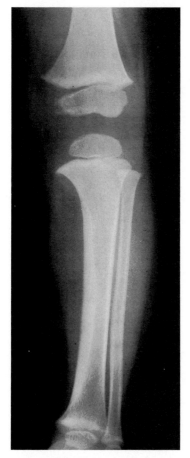

Figure 3–99 Normal leg, 2 years.

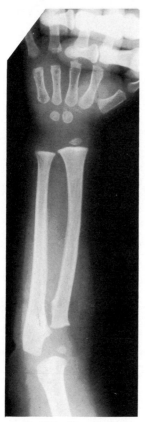

Figure 3–100 Normal forearm.

Answers

Patricia Plumb's bones show a very wide, very dense transverse line in the metaphysis, the location of which corresponds to the normally somewhat dense zone of provisional calcification seen in a normal growing bone. (Compare with Figure 3–99.) Ingested metallic lead interferes with the process of replacement of provisionally calcified bars of cartilage by endosteal bone, resulting in a disc of compact calcified cartilage which grows thicker as long as environmental exposure to lead continues. Although a small amount of lead is deposited in the same region, it is not sufficient to result in a significant increase in roentgen density. Patricia's diagnosis was confirmed by a serum lead determination.

After much questioning of *Billy Johnson's* parents you discover that he is left with his elderly grandmother for a long weekend occasionally. This good woman, convinced that the child was undernourished, dosed him heavily from a large and ancient bottle of phosphorylated cod liver oil. The dense metaphyseal bands caused by ingestion of phosphorus are indistinguishable from those caused by lead. Pathologically, they are quite different, however. Phosphorus poisoning results in an increased number of true bony trabeculae in the metaphyseal spongiosa. We show you this case because it illustrates the way in which the metaphysis of a bone provides us with a record of what has been happening to bone growth in recent months. Here, the *distance between* the dense bands is a "marked" index to the rate of growth: obviously the distal radius and ulna are growing much more rapidly than the distal humerus!

In Figure 3–101, you see *Ricky Stump's* leg many weeks later following treatment with vitamin D. In the active phase of rickets, the growth plate continues to proliferate, forming masses of cartilage that, because of lack of calcium, fail to mineralize. Widening of the radiolucent growth plate results (compare in Figure 3–97 directly with the same area in Figure 3–101). The dense zone of provisional calcification fails to visualize on the radiograph. Without the strength afforded by calcification, the poorly formed cartilage and the osteoid matrix laid down upon it by continued activity of osteoblasts are compressed laterally by weight bearing, and flaring of the metaphysis results. Impaction of the epiphysis into the weakened growing area results in the characteristic cupping (seen best in Ricky's ankle). Bone in the shaft continues to undergo normal turnover but is replaced with unmineralized osteoid, resulting in loss of rigidity and subsequent bowing.

It is an interesting fact of bone metabolism that osteoclastic destruction of osteoid cannot take place unless that osteoid has been mineralized. Thus, the accumulation of uncalcified osteoid matrix also accounts for the radiolucency and modeling failure seen here (Fig. 3–101). Note that the bowing of the shaft has been impressively corrected.

In contrast to rickets (which is osteomalacia of growing bone), vitamin C deficiency results in the osteoporotic condition of scurvy, seen in *Mina See.* Vitamin C is essential to the normal production of osteoid (collagen plus ground substance) by osteoblasts. Without it there is a reduced rate of proliferation of the cartilage cells of the growth plate as well. Because there is no disturbance of deposition of calcium salts in cartilage, however, the zone of provisional calcification thickens and increases in density. This gives rise to the "white line of scurvy," seen on radiographs at the very end of the metaphysis. The calcified cartilage thus formed is weak and subject to many small infractions, resulting in irregularity of its roentgen image. (Contrast this with the smooth, wider dense line of lead poisoning.)

On the diaphyseal side of this line there is a zone of lucency where previously formed spongy bone of the metaphysis is undergoing resorption, but it is not being revised or replaced. Severe *osteoporosis* is the result. You have probably noted the tibial subperiosteal hemorrhages (beginning to calcify), also a common occurrence in this disease. They are due both to capillary fragility and to the many small fractures of the metaphysis. In scurvy you may even see a gross fracture through the zone of metaphyseal osteoporosis with marked displacement of the epiphysis.

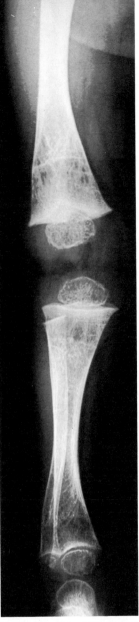

Figure 3–101 Ricky's leg many weeks later after treatment with vitamin D.

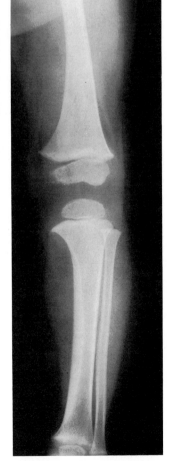

Figure 3–102 Normal leg.

Part D

Bone on Your Own

Introduction

The material in the first three sections of this workbook has been conscientiously gathered into groups of *related* problems in an attempt to make specific clinical ideas clear. We will now abandon this arrangement for a series of unrelated problems in bone diagnosis, much as you might see them during the course of your rotation in the emergency room.

As before, pertinent clinical data will be provided and, just as a good medical history does, will often supply diagnostic clues. It is our avowed tendency (and delight) to make these data provocative—but in doing so we may (as may any of your patients) lead you down the path to an erroneous "snap" diagnosis. You may guard against this by first making a careful inspection in an *organized* way of the entire film, just as you have learned to do with films of the chest and abdomen. We suggest that you make the following systematic observations in each of the cases in the remainder of this book— and those that you encounter in real life.

1. *Overall size and shape:* Are these consistent with the patient's age and sex? If on the film obtained you have a *series* of bones—fingers, ribs, vertebrae—does any one bone not fit into the progression?

2. *Local size and shape:* Are there any unusual narrowings or protuberances?

3. *Thickness of cortex:* In a long bone, is it normally thick at midshaft, gradually becoming thinner at the flaring metaphysis? In a round bone, is it visible all the way around?

4. *Trabecular pattern:* Are trabeculae present in normal numbers? Normally spaced? Well or poorly defined? Thickened? Thinned? Arrangement altered?

5. *General density of the whole bone:* Increased or decreased?

6. *Local density change:* If so, increased or decreased? Solitary or multiple?

7. *Margination of local lesions:* Sharp and well-defined? Is there a surrounding zone of increased density? Or poorly defined and fading gradually into the surrounding bony substance?

8. *Break in continuity:* Particularly of the cortex in profile.

9. *Periosteal change:* If present, is it dense (hard)? Lacy (soft)? Layered? Spiculated?

10. *Soft tissue change:* Localized mass? Calcification? Reduced muscle mass? Foreign body?

Of course, this list does not cover all possibilities, but if you can reach a reasoned conclusion about each of the ten categories, always using the normal for comparison, you will certainly be able to arrive at a good many diagnoses without help.

Problems

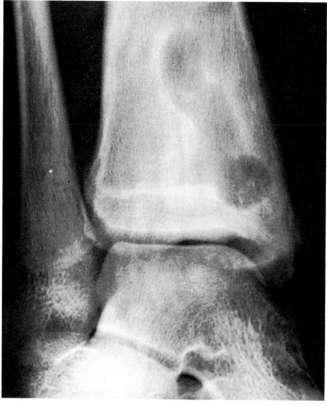

Figure 3–103 Kevin Farrell

Kevin Farrell, age 20, is complaining of dull pain in his ankle, present for several weeks. There is no history of injury. After discovering that his temperature is 38.3°C and his white blood cell count is 18,750, you order the film seen here. Closer questioning reveals that he had a superficial abscess of his calf treated by incision and drainage over three months ago.

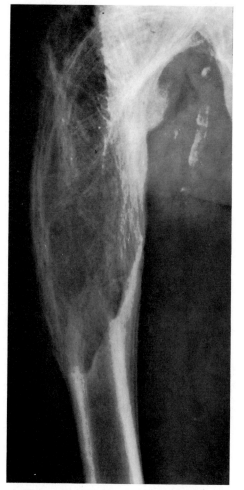

Figure 3–104 Harvey Immergluck

Harvey Immergluck, retired, has hip pain. On physical examination his prostate is smoothly enlarged and firm. Your work-up includes an ultrasound-guided prostate biopsy, which shows benign prostatic hypertrophy, and plain films of the painful hip and proximal femur. A radiograph of that bone is seen here.

Jenny Dowben, age nine, has a long history of multiple fractures, particularly of her left lower extremity, occurring usually after minor trauma. She is brought to the emergency room, this time because of sudden pain in the left leg just below the knee. Your attention is drawn to her eyes, which have sclerae of a definite blue color.

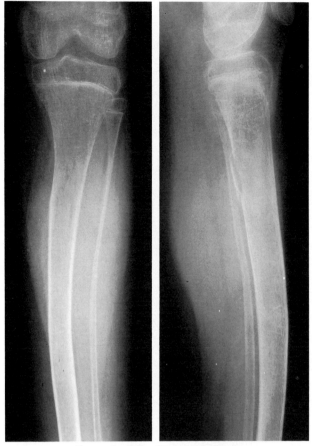

Figure 3–105 Jenny Dowben

Raffaello Sanzio is five years old. He is severely anemic and his liver and spleen are enlarged. You learn from his parents that his older sister died six years ago of a "blood disease."

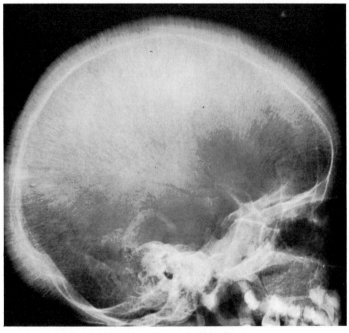

Figure 3–106 Raffaello Sanzio

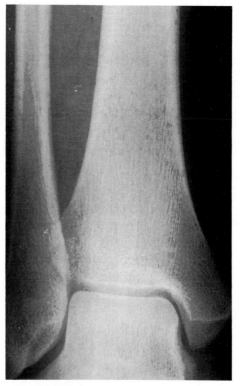

Figure 3–107 Normal.

Answers

When you first look at the bones in this film of *Mr. Farrell's* ankle, you see only a curious localized decrease in density and some evidence of early cortical destruction along the medial aspect of the tibial metaphysis. Closer examination makes it possible to decide that there is definite loss of cortex in the same region as the periosteal change. You could describe the lucency as well defined, with a slightly sclerotic border, and serpiginous in shape, which is not at all suggestive of a tumor growing centrifugally.

The historical facts suggest an inflammatory lesion of bone, and the film is an excellent example of typical hematogenous osteomyelitis. Predilection for the metaphysis is classic and is related to the anatomy of the blood supply to the region.

Mr. Immergluck's benign prostatic hypertrophy has nothing whatever to do with his femur. There is a marked localized increase in size of the bone and abnormality of the cortex, thickening, and a loss of density and uniformity. The trabeculae are reduced in numbers and appear disorganized and individually thickened. The sharply defined and rather angular zone of demarcation from the normal bone of the distal shaft is in contrast to the impression of an expanding process seen proximally. There is laminated periosteal new bone medially, but there is no localized bone destruction anywhere. Disorder of bony structure and general expansion of bone without any localized destruction are the findings that distinguish Paget's disease from tumor.

Bone changes like those you see here are often found to progress to the more typical changes of Paget's disease like those in Figure 3–8, and now three stages of the disease are recognized: (1) destructive; (2) reparative; (3) and quiescent.

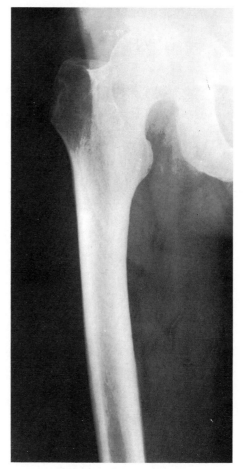

Figure 3–108 Normal.

A history such as *Jenny Dowben's* can mean only one diagnosis—the disease formerly (and graphically) known as *fragilitas ossium,* now more explicitly termed *osteogenesis imperfecta.* The defect of collagen formation (thus, also of bone matrix) is inherited as a dominant trait. Fortunately, it is rare. An occasional affected individual survives intrauterine life, the traumas of birth, and the immediate postpartum period, with appearance of extreme bony fragility later in infancy and childhood.

The bones of Jenny's leg show roentgen changes typical of osteoporosis. In her case the osteoporosis resulting from the bone-producing defect has been accentuated by immobilization for earlier healing fractures. Her most recent symptoms are related to the posterior cortical fracture near the knee. Note the extreme attenuation of the fibular shaft.

(Blue sclerae are also related to deficiency in collagen production. The extremely thin, and thus somewhat translucent, sclerae allow the dark pigment of the choroid to show through.)

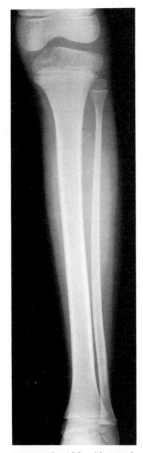

Figure 3–109 Normal.

The film you obtained on *Raffaello Sanzio* is very abnormal. The calvarium is enlarged and the abnormality involves all the bones equally. The inner cortex (or table) is normal but the outer is difficult to identify. Where the x-ray beam is tangential to it, you have the impression of a brush (or "hair-on-end") appearance. In other areas these are projected differently. The history suggests this child is suffering from a hereditary blood disorder. Your laboratory studies confirm the diagnosis of thalassemia major. The appearance of the skull is due to the marked hyperplasia of bone marrow.

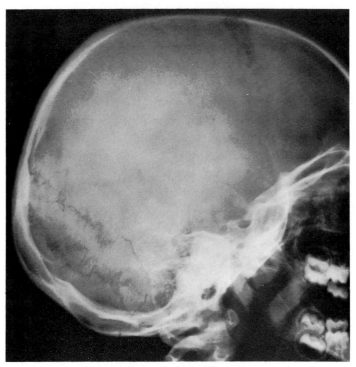

Figure 3–110 Normal.

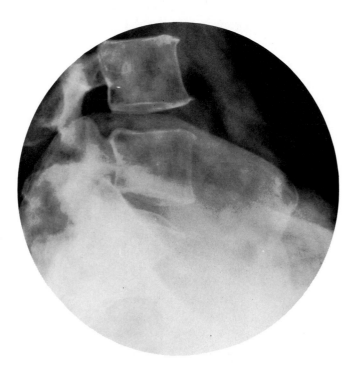

Figure 3–111   Mr. Cecil Northrup

Problems

Cecil Northrup, 67 years old, is a retired bank president. He is complaining of lower abdominal distention, urinary frequency, and vague back pain. Your physical examination reveals a distended bladder and an enlarged prostate. In the course of his work-up, an IVU was done. Changes in the bones seen on that study lead to a skeletal survey of which the film shown is a part.

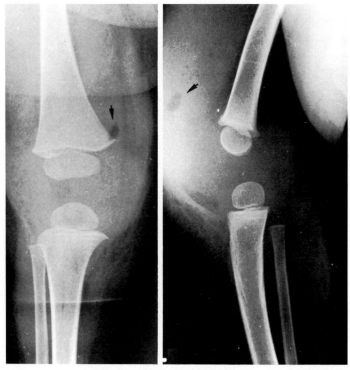

Figure 3–112   Carlos Rigsby

Carlos Rigsby, age one, is brought in by his parents, who state that for the past three days he has screamed in apparent pain whenever his diaper was changed. Yesterday Mrs. Rigsby was able to localize this to his right knee because of the appearance of massive swelling. You note several furuncles on his back and arms, which his mother has been treating with "poultices." His temperature is 39.4°C and the white blood cell count is 20,285.

Sharon Lippitt is a 14-year-old girl with hysterical tendencies. She is brought (or one might almost say dragged) in by her angry mother, who says that Sharon will not practice for a forthcoming piano recital. After you have gently removed the mother from the examining room, Sharon becomes calmer, but she insists that her shoulder has been bothering her for over six months, particularly when she is playing the piano. X-ray films were made four months ago and showed nothing abnormal. Your examination reveals only some limitation of motion and moderate tenderness over the head of the humerus.

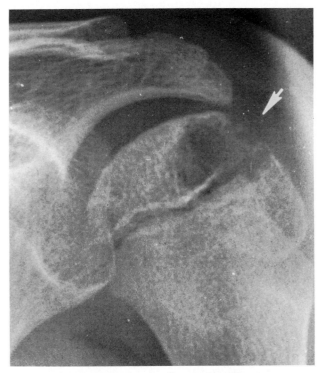

Figure 3–113 Sharon Lippitt

Henry Sturdevant, six years old, is brought in after having fallen out of an apple tree. He is complaining of shoulder pain.

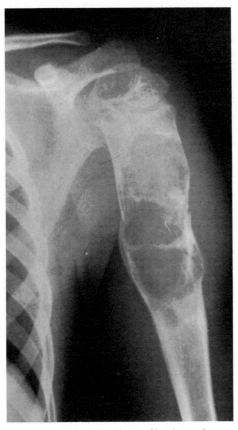

Figure 3–114 Henry Sturdevant

Page 237

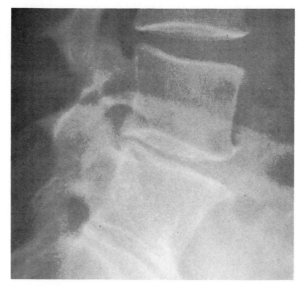

Figure 3–115 Normal (except for the disc).

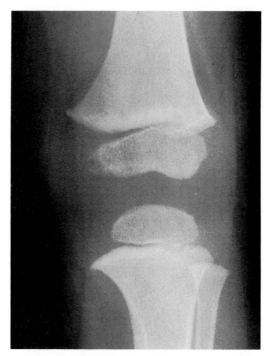

Figure 3–116 Normal.

Answers

The multiple discrete areas of increased bone density seen in *Mr. Northrup's* pelvis and lower lumbar spine are metastases from his unsuspected carcinoma of the prostate, proved by prostatic biopsy. This example is considerably more subtle than those you have seen previously. Only a careful inspection for uniformity of bone density will reveal the presence of the lesions.

Seventy per cent of patients with carcinoma of the prostate will show evidence at some time of metastasis to bone. The lumbar spine and pelvis are involved with greater frequency. The mode of spread of prostatic carcinoma was explained in 1940 by Batson, whose name is now forever attached to his discovery. He was able to demonstrate communication between the venous plexus surrounding the prostate and that draining the sacrum, ilia, and lumbar spine. He showed that blood flow was toward the spine in the recumbent position and in the opposite direction in the upright posture.

Carlos Rigsby shows no bony changes in his knee at this time. There is marked distension of the knee joint, however, resulting in separation of the femur from the tibia. The small lucency indicated by the arrow is gas produced by the infecting organism in this example of septic arthritis. Findings such as this in a joint are a true emergency. Prompt specific therapy, including drainage of purulent material from the joint and high doses of antibiotics, will be necessary if the integrity of the joint is to be preserved. Unfortunately, many patients with septic arthritis have extensive cartilage destruction by the time they are treated, and the joint becomes ankylosed.

Sharon Lippitt has a purely destructive process of the epiphysis of the humerus. It is also beginning to erode across the growth plate to involve the metaphysis. The most striking finding is the absence of any sclerosis or other reparative response by the surrounding bone. The location of the lesion at the edge of the articular cartilage of the humeral head is notable. During the course of her hospital studies, a positive tuberculin test is discovered. It had previously been negative, according to school records. This, then, is an example of tuberculous osteomyelitis. Contrast it with the pyogenic osteomyelitis in Figure 3–103 and review the differences in the findings.

Henry Sturdevant has an unsuspected lytic lesion of the proximal humerus, leading to pathologic fracture. A close look will reveal interruptions in the markedly thinned bony cortex about the midpoint of the lesion. A destructive expanding lesion such as this, occurring at the metaphyseal end of a long bone in a young person, is most likely to be a so-called "unicameral" cyst of bone. The facts of the patient's age and that the lesion stops short of the growth plate help to differentiate it from giant cell tumor, which this example otherwise resembles. Giant cell tumors are usually seen in mature bones.

The ultimate diagnosis of tumorous conditions of bone therefore depends on accumulation of data, not all of which are related to the roentgen appearance of the lesion. Age, sex, sites of predilection, and other specific historical data as well as the x-ray appearance of the lesion all seem to narrow the list of possibilities and ultimately allow a histologic diagnosis.

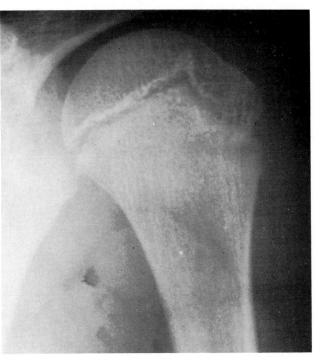

Figure 3–117 Normal.

Problems

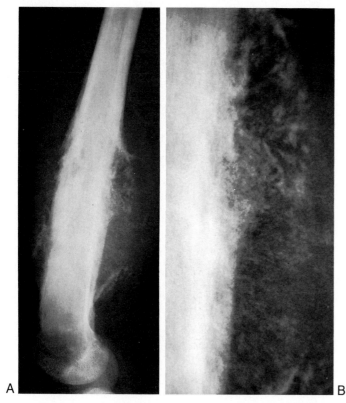

Figure 3–118 Thomas Stanton. **A,** Full view. **B,** Detail.

Thomas Stanton is a 27-year-old machinist whose tolerance for standing at his job has been steadily decreasing because of pain in his right thigh. Up to this time he has ignored a tender swelling just above the knee. He comes for medical help only because he has been threatened with dismissal from his job.

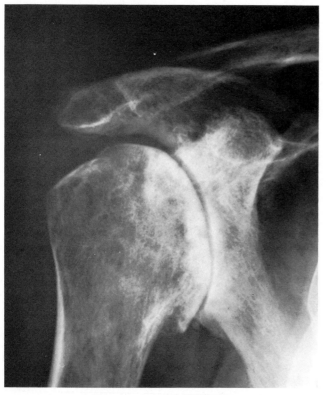

Figure 3–119 Elmer Davis

Elmer Davis is a 65-year-old retired seaman who is complaining of pain and stiffness in both shoulders, more severe on the right. Otherwise he is well.

Belle Thistlethwaite is a left-handed painter who has been treating her swollen right wrist with hot compresses for three weeks while trying to complete a portrait.

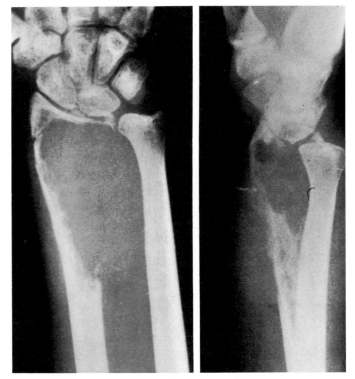

Figure 3–120 Belle Thistlethwaite

Henrietta Hobson, age 25, a nurse in the coronary care unit, appears often at the hospital emergency room for treatment of episodes of severe abdominal pain and anemia. Her family history reveals that two other siblings have a similar problem. The film shown here was made because of a complaint of pain in the upper arm.

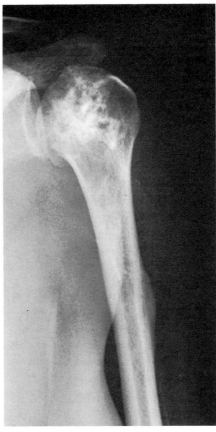

Figure 3–121 Henrietta Hobson

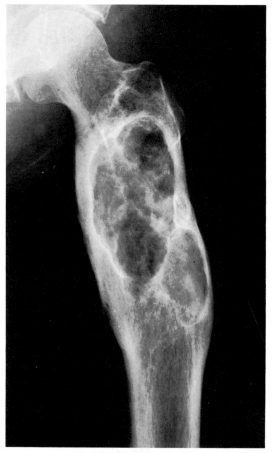

Figure 3–122 Mr. Gardner

Mr. Gardner, age 45, has had a dull aching pain in the left hip for about two years. Today, during a game of touch football, he was kicked in the thigh and comes in complaining of a "charleyhorse."

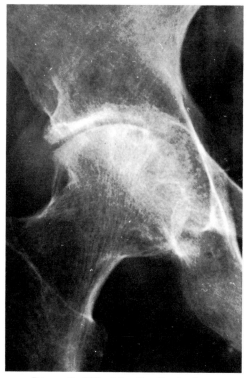

Figure 3–123 Mrs. Heatherington

Mrs. Heatherington, age 50, has been ill for 20 years with severe "rheumatism." Both hips have been painful and limited in range of motion, and her hands have also been stiff and painful. Today she fell in the bathtub and complains of an unusual amount of pain in her right hip.

Mrs. O'Flaherty, 68 years old, was running to catch a bus; as she stepped off the curb, she fell, with sudden severe pain in her left hip. As she lies on a stretcher, you note external rotation of her left foot and some shortening of the left lower extremity.

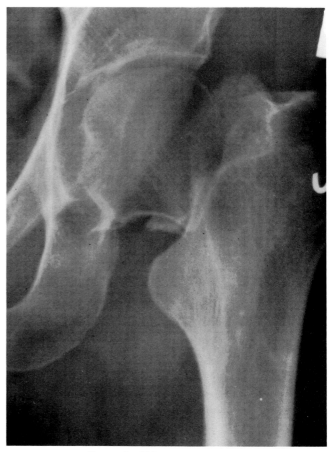

Figure 3–124 Mrs. O'Flaherty

Jamie Holloway, four years old, has been complaining of pain in his left leg for ten days. He skinned his knee three weeks ago and it appears to be infected. He refuses to walk or stand, appears toxic, and has a fever of 39.4°C. Complete blood count shows a leukocytosis of 24,000.

1. In which patient(s) is trauma the sole cause of the hip pain?
2. In which might trauma be partly responsible for the changes seen?
3. In which is there osteoporosis that you can be sure of?
4. In which is the hip joint itself abnormal?
5. If you think any of these patients has a tumor, does it appear to be benign or malignant?

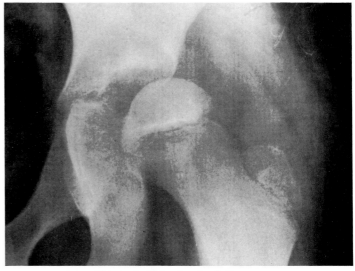

Figure 3–125 Jamie Holloway

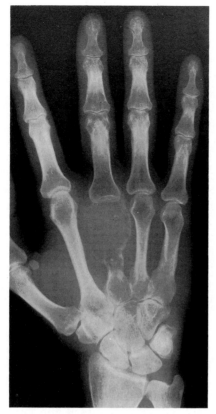

Figure 3–129 Mrs. H.

Final Exercise (Bones of Contention)

It is not only gypsy fortune-tellers who find hands of great interest in predicting the future. Radiologists and other specialists have often been impressed with the frequency with which radiographs of the hands reflect a generalized disease process. In addition, the human hand, because it is the marvelous evolutionary tool that it is, constantly gets itself into machines, under saws and hammers, and into other unhealthy places. Hands radiographed after trauma often show evidence of some other disease condition not yet diagnosed.

The hand films on this and the next several pages should be examined in sequence and your impressions noted on scrap paper. A normal film is included, and once you decide which it is, it will be useful to you as a guide. A series of descriptions follows on page 253. These are to be answered by entering the appropriate patient's initial in the blank following each question. Correctly filled in, the answers will spell (vertically) what we'll do with you as you close the book.

Mrs. H is a 35-year-old woman who has noted swelling in the midportion of her hand that was painless until a few hours ago. She experienced sudden pain in this area while attempting to open a seldom-used pancake syrup bottle.

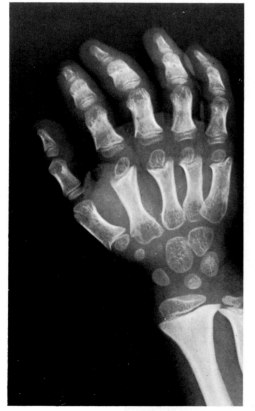

Figure 3–130 Master E.

Master E is six years old and much shorter than he should be for his age. His parents, who are of average height, are concerned.

This elderly man, *Mr. A,* has been a manual laborer for many years. In the past six or seven years he has had recurrent episodes of severe pain in the fingers, brought on by exposure to cold. He is no longer able to flex his fingers. The skin of his hands is shiny, pale, and indurated.

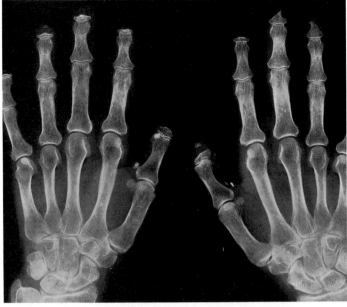

Figure 3–131 Mr. A.

Master K is three years old and has fractured his tibia without apparent trauma. The hand film is part of a skeletal survey.

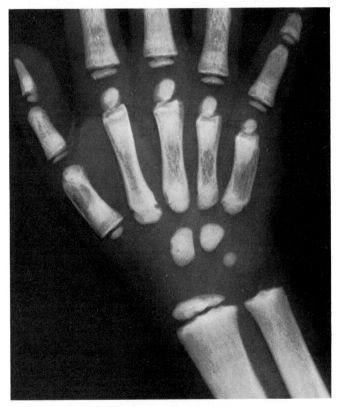

Figure 3–132 Master K.

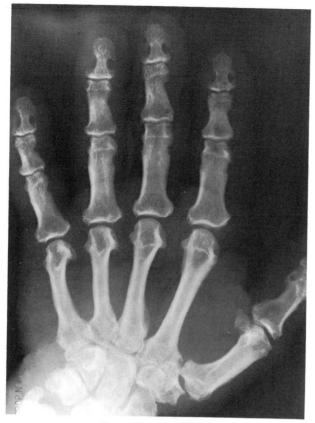

Figure 3–137   Mr. N.

Mr. N is 32 years old and comes to you because last winter's hat and gloves, at that time a perfect fit, are now extremely small for him. His wife also has noted a great change in his facial appearance, particularly after comparison with last summer's snapshots.

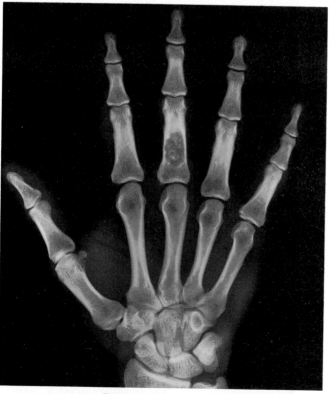

Figure 3–138   Mr. D.

Mr. D caught his fingers in a car door. There is no external sign of injury when you examine him, but because he is complaining bitterly you request just this one view of the hand.

Instructions, Questions, and Acrostic

The game here is to find a patient to fit each of the roentgen descriptions below. Enter that patient's initial in the blank to the left. You may not actually use all the illustrations. Several patients are described more than once.

_____ 1. THERE IS A PATCHY LOSS OF SPONGIOSA AND CORTICAL THINNING IN ALL THE BONES, CONSISTENT WITH SEVERE OSTEOPOROSIS. THERE IS ALSO MARKED NARROWING AND DESTRUCTION OF THE DISTAL INTERPHALANGEAL JOINTS.

_____ 2. THE BONES ARE GENERALLY TOO SHORT, BUT THE MIDSHAFT DIAMETER IS NORMAL.

_____ 3. A DISEASE OF KINGS AND OTHER HIGH LIVERS.

_____ 4. THERE ARE THREE AREAS OF LOCALIZED SOFT TISSUE SWELLING, WITH DESTRUCTION OF UNDERLYING BONE.

_____ 5. THERE ARE IRREGULAR EROSIONS OF THE HEADS OF THE METACARPALS AND ALSO OF THE CARPAL BONES.

_____ 6. THERE IS A SOLITARY, LYTIC, MODERATELY RAPIDLY GROWING TUMOR.

_____ 7. THERE IS PERIARTICULAR SOFT TISSUE CALCIFICATION.

_____ 8. THERE IS GENERALIZED INCREASE IN DENSITY OF ALL THE BONES.

_____ 9. THERE IS A CONGENITAL DEFECT OF CARTILAGE PROLIFERATION IN GROWING BONE.

_____ 10. A SOLITARY LESION HAS EXPANDED THE CORTEX UNTIL IT IS ONLY A THIN SHELL, IN PLACES NOT VISIBLE.

_____ 11. THERE HAS BEEN ABSORPTION OF THE TUFTS OF ALL DISTAL PHALANGES.

_____ 12. THERE IS NOTABLE INCREASE IN SOFT TISSUE THICKNESS, GENERALLY. THE BONES ARE NORMAL IN LENGTH BUT INCREASED IN DIAMETER.

_____ 13. A SOLITARY, DEFINITELY BENIGN LESION.

_____ 14. THERE IS ABSENCE OF THE ULNAR STYLOID PROCESS AND INVOLVEMENT OF METACARPOPHALANGEAL JOINTS BUT LITTLE CHANGE ABOUT THE INTERPHALANGEAL JOINTS.

Answers

(Do not read until you have completed the exercise.)

Mrs. H has a rather aggressive-looking solitary lesion; microscopically it proved to be a malignant giant cell tumor. From its roentgen appearance, because it has eroded the cortex completely in places, one cannot be sure that it is benign. There may be a pathologic fracture present, although such fractures occur in bone weakened by either benign or malignant tumors. The precise diagnosis here would not be known until after the surgical excision and microscopic study, but the radiographic appearance would suggest that the lesion is malignant.

Master E is an achondroplastic dwarf.

Mr. A has a condition known as sclerodactyly, which is related to the collagen diseases—progressive systemic sclerosis (scleroderma), which this patient ultimately proved to have. There is often periarticular soft tissue calcification.

Master K clearly has osteopetrosis. We have seen a case earlier in this volume. This one presents the interesting "bone within a bone" appearance seen in patients with this condition. It is thought to be due to transient amelioration of the inborn defect for a short time during active growth of the bone.

Mrs. O's hand film is, of course, normal. (Can glass be seen on radiographs?)

Miss S has advanced rheumatoid arthritis. The other cardinal features (in addition to those referred to in the acrostic) are juxta-articular osteoporosis and joint narrowing and destruction. The causes of osteoporosis in this disease are many. Acutely, it is usually juxta-articular and caused by increased vascularity about the inflamed joints. Later, with severe deformity, osteoporosis occurs because of disuse. Steroid therapy also results in generalized osteoporosis because of the catabolic effects of the hormone on bone. Could this also explain the history of gastrointestinal hemorrhage?

Mrs. W has degenerative joint disease of multiple small joints of the hands. There is thinning of joint cartilage and proliferative change (the addition of new bone, osteophytes, at the margins of the joints)—characteristically at the distal interphalangeal joints. This gives rise to the hard juxta-articular nodules known as Heberden's nodes. *Mrs. W* also has Sudeck's posttraumatic atrophy.

Mr. L is suffering from an inherited defect of purine metabolism, resulting in the clinical syndrome of gouty arthritis. The etiology of arthritis in gout is not entirely clear but seems to be related to the deposition of uric acid crystals in periarticular soft tissues. The typical changes of moderately advanced disease are seen here, with sharply gouged-out destructive lesions of juxta-articular bone. There is no tendency toward symmetry, as in rheumatoid arthritis. Note also that there is no apparent loss of articular cartilage as one would see in rheumatoid and degenerative arthritis.

Mr. N is suffering from the effects on adult bone of excessive secretion of pituitary growth hormone, probably by an eosinophilic adenoma of the pituitary. Because the epiphyses are fused, growth in length is not possible. Growth in diameter as the result of excessive periosteal bone deposition occurs. The soft tissues are also stimulated and become thicker in acromegaly. These patients have marked coarsening of facial features, with prominence of the eyebrows, forehead, and jaw. Note that overproduction of bone has resulted in bridging between distal phalangeal tufts and shafts.

Mr. D has a small, benign enchondroma of his third proximal phalanx. It was found, as so many of them are, incidentally. They occasionally become large enough to make the bone prone to pathologic fracture. Note the characteristic calcification within the lesion.

(Now, turn the page for the answer to the acrostic.)

Now - - - - - - -

W
E
'
L
L

S
H
A
K
E

H
A
N
D
S
!

CONTENTS

To use this chapter properly, always begin with the historical vignette in Part A. Decide on film findings, appropriate procedures, and management before going on to each new part. Then thumb to the next part and specific page by referring to the notation in bold type on the right margin of each right-hand page.

The division into parts has been done with the specific purpose of forcing the reader to pause before seeing the answers. If the system described here is used, the reader should be able to move from one section to another within five seconds.

The cases are arranged to reflect the wide variety of clinical problems that arise daily and randomly.

Part A

TWO PATIENTS WITH FLU SYMPTOMS

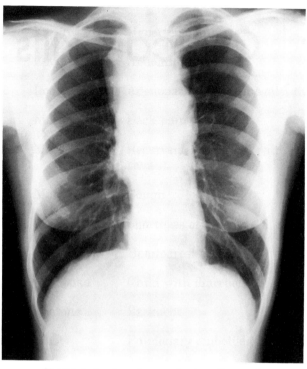

Figure 4–1 Amy Long, chest radiograph.

Amy Long, a 22-year-old college student, was sent to you by the college infirmary for evaluation of a right neck mass and flu-like symptoms of several weeks' duration. She had a chest film taken at the infirmary (Fig. 4–1), and it is available for your evaluation. On physical examination, you find a fever of 100° F, a 2 × 2 cm firm right anterior cervical mass, and an enlarged spleen. What diagnosis are you considering? What do you think of the chest film?

Continued Part B, page 278.

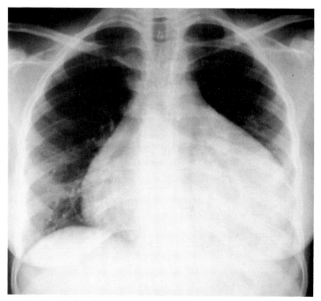

Figure 4–2 Juliana Clementine, chest radiograph.

Juliana Clementine, a previously healthy 19-year-old piano student, is sent to your emergency department by her university health service with a flu-like syndrome of several days' duration and an abnormal chest film. See Figure 4–2. What do you think of this chest radiograph? What are the possible diagnoses?

Continued Part B, page 278.

THREE PATIENTS WITH COUGH

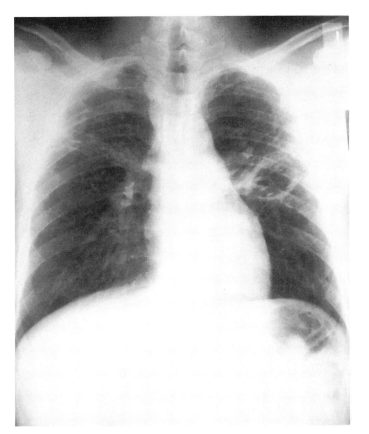

Figure 4–3 John Doe, PA chest radiograph.

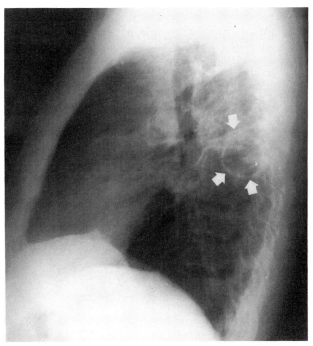

Figure 4–4 Mr. Doe, lateral chest radiograph.

A middle-aged man comes to your emergency department with cough and fever of several weeks' duration and vague back pain. He appears disheveled, with numerous needle track marks along his upper extremities suggesting extensive short- and long-term intravenous drug use. He refuses to give you his name. On physical examination, you find **"Mr. Doe"** to have a temperature of 100° F, but there are no other positive findings relating to the heart and lungs. His WBC is 9000 with 50% lymphocytes. You also note a significant alcoholic odor about him. Figures 4–3 and 4–4 are the PA and lateral chest films that you obtain in the emergency department. What do you think? What diagnosis are you going to consider?

Continued Part B, page 279.

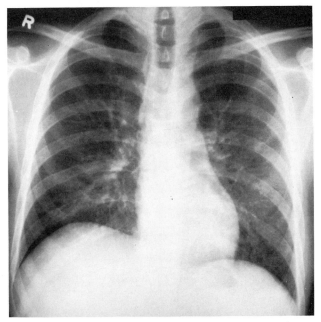

Figure 4–5 Brian Seldinger, PA chest radiograph.

Brian Seldinger, a 31-year-old father of two and bicycle salesman and enthusiast, comes to your emergency department with a dry, hacking, nonproductive cough of several days' duration, dyspnea, and low-grade fever. He has never smoked. What do you think of his PA chest radiograph taken in the emergency room (Fig. 4–5)?

Continued Part B, page 279.

Jeff Stitson, a 32-year-old chief neurology resident, grabs you in the hall and tells you that he has had acute chest pain, high fever, and cough with sputum for several days. You quickly whisk him into a nearby examining room and find on physical examination significantly diminished breath sounds in the left upper lung field poste-riorly. Because you are the chief resident in medicine, he trusts your judgment, and based upon your physical findings he wants you to put him on antibiotics. You convince him of the need for a chest film. You take him down to the radiology department and get PA and lateral views of the chest. What do you think? Look at Figures 4–6 and 4–7.

Continued Part B, page 280.

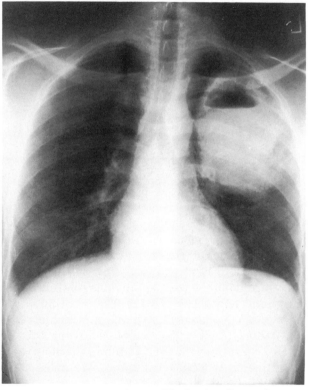

Figure 4–6 Jeff Stitson, PA chest radiograph.

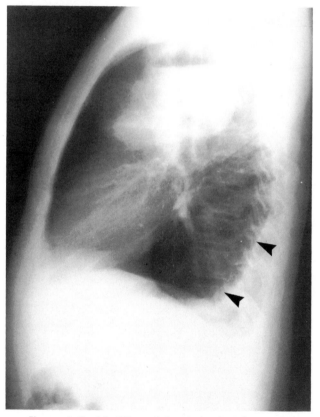

Figure 4–7 Mr. Stitson, lateral chest radiograph.

PATIENT WITH SHORTNESS OF BREATH (SOB)

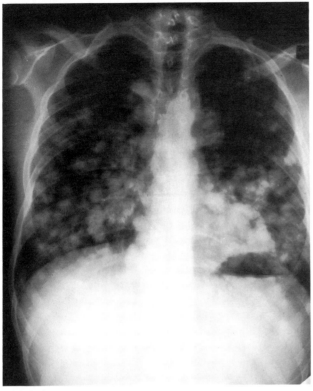

Paul O'Grady, a 43-year-old baseball card dealer, comes to your clinic with complaints of increasing shortness of breath over the past three weeks. He is afebrile and reports no other symptoms. He has no history of heart disease. He never smoked and denies any history of pulmonary problems. What do you think of his initial PA chest film (Fig. 4–8)? What will you do next?

Continued Part B, page 280.

Figure 4–8 Paul O'Grady, PA chest radiograph.

PATIENT WITH ACUTE BACK PAIN

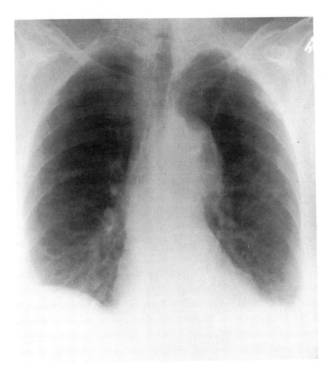

Matilda Mason, a 60-year-old woman, came to your emergency department complaining of severe acute back pain in the thoracic region. On physical examination, you find an elderly, pale woman in severe pain. Her blood pressure is normal and she has a slightly elevated temperature of 101° F. Laboratory data are unremarkable, except for Hb of 11 g. You obtain a chest radiograph (Fig. 4–9). What do you think?

Continued Part B, page 280.

Figure 4–9 Matilda Mason, chest radiograph.

THREE PATIENTS WITH DIARRHEA

Lisa Morgan, age 23, arrives at the hospital with a temperature of 37.5° C, complaining of diarrhea, nausea, and right lower quadrant pain. On questioning it seems her complaints are actually of two weeks' duration and that this is her third similar episode in five months. Last summer she had her first attack of sharp, intermittent right lower quadrant pain and several loose bowel movements unassociated with meals or activity. She ran a low-grade fever. Her symptoms lasted seven days and then gradually abated. A month later, she had another attack of right lower quadrant pain, diarrhea, and evening temperature elevation. X-ray studies of the gastrointestinal (GI) tract and colon were negative, and blood studies were normal. She again improved after a week.

At present she appears pale and somewhat thin for her build. Blood studies show white blood count (WBC) 12,000, hemoglobin (Hb) 10.1, hematocrit (Hct) 32. The serum albumin is decreased and the corrected sedimentation rate is 60. Urinalysis is negative. On physical examination there is a 10-cm area of fullness in the right lower quadrant that is very tender to palpation. Rectal examination reveals a tender fullness in the right vault. Hyperextension of the right leg elicits deep right lower quadrant pain.

What imaging studies would you request? You primarily suspect inflammatory bowel disease or, less likely, appendicitis.

Continued Part B, page 281.

John Gaunt, 28, has been in the hospital for ten days under treatment for ulcerative colitis. His disease was first diagnosed when he was a senior in college. Except for occasional exacerbations characterized by periods of abdominal cramps, diarrhea, and rectal bleeding, he has done well on low maintenance dosage of antibiotics. Now hospitalized because of a recent flare-up, he was responding to prednisone and increased antibiotic therapy until two days ago.

Since then his condition has deteriorated, with alarming increase in abdominal pain, cramps, and bloody diarrhea. This morning his temperature has climbed to 40.6° C, and there has been a massive outpouring of blood from the rectum. On physical examination, his abdomen is markedly distended, exquisitely tender, and silent to auscultation. You request a film of the abdomen and also consider an emergency barium enema to see what has gone wrong. Here is the plain film of the abdomen (Fig. 4–10).

Continued Part B, page 281.

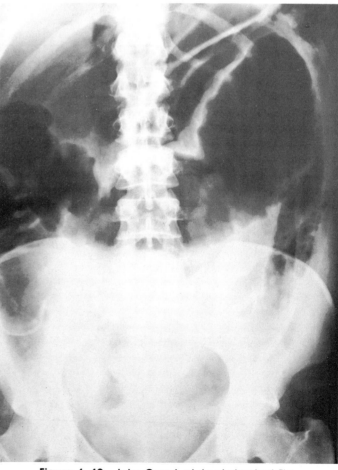

Figure 4–10 John Gaunt, plain abdominal film.

Pierre Claude, 56, the noted chef de cuisine from Juan-les-Pins, is forced to interrupt his lecture tour and enter the hospital. He tells you he has been suffering from diarrhea for the past week, three to four semisolid stools a day with a great deal of mucus but no blood. He consulted a doctor in another city who believed Monsieur Claude's symptoms were due to a strenuous tour schedule and the change from his usual diet. Yesterday the patient began to have crampy lower abdominal pain. He gave himself an enema, which was productive of a small amount of fecal material but no gas. The pain steadily increased in severity; his abdomen became distended and tense; and he consulted another physician, who recommended admission to the hospital.

On physical examination, there is moderate abdominal tenderness and you can palpate dilated bowel in the left upper and lower quadrants. High-pitched tinkles are heard in the abdomen on auscultation. T 37.5° C; BP 145/80; P 90; WBC 7300.

What x-ray examination would you request?

Continued Part B, page 282.

THREE PATIENTS WITH RUQ PAIN

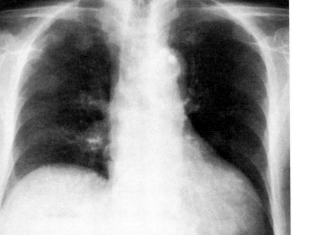

Figure 4-11   Agnes Delarenzo, PA chest radiograph

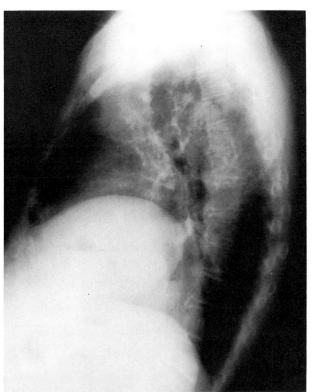

Figure 4-12   Mrs. Delarenzo, lateral chest radiograph.

Agnes Delarenzo, a 69-year-old woman, came to your emergency department with excruciating right upper abdominal pain, fever, malaise, and shaking chills. On physical examination you find an elderly, shaking, ill-appearing woman with a temperature of 103° F, BP of 110/70, and exquisite tenderness in the right upper abdomen by the anterior rib cage. Figures 4–11 and 4–12 are the initial posteroanterior (PA) and lateral chest films. What do you think?

Continued Part B, page 282.

Leo Cleveland, a previously healthy 55-year-old furniture salesman, comes to your office with a two-week history of right upper quadrant pain, which has become more epigastric in location over the last few days. On physical examination, you notice dullness to percussion over the left lower chest and upper abdominal tenderness. The amylase level is reported to be 7800. His chest film confirmed a left pleural effusion as the cause of his left chest dullness on physical examination (Fig. 4–13). What diagnosis are you considering? What imaging tests would you request?

Continued Part B, page 283.

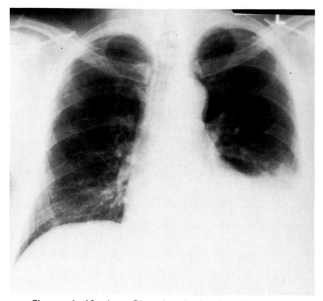

Figure 4–13 Leo Cleveland, chest radiograph.

Harvey Conrad, a 43-year-old overweight electrician, comes to your office complaining of right upper abdominal pain that has bothered him intermittently over the past year. The pain is often accompanied by dyspepsia, with belching, nausea, and flatulence. Mr. Conrad avoids eating fatty foods because they do not agree with him. He has been previously healthy without prior gastrointestinal complaints. His physical examination is unremarkable, and the stool is guaiac negative. He denies fever or jaundice. How will you work up Mr. Conrad?

Continued Part B, page 283.

TWO PATIENTS WITH GI BLEED

Jacques de Gautière, 20, college student, is brought to the emergency ward of your hospital after he fainted in class this morning. He tells you he has been in no pain of any kind but did pass a large black stool yesterday. He is in apparent excellent general health except for some pallor and understandable anxiety. He has never been seen in clinic before. Vital signs are normal except for postural hypotension, but the Hct is 28 and the stool black and 4+ guaiac positive. What should you do first?

Continued Part B, page 284.

Abner Lane, a 78-year-old florist, was well until three hours ago, when he passed a large amount of bright red blood following his morning bowel movement. He has been passing small amounts of blood with clots nearly every 20 minutes since then. Mr. Lane has always been in good health and this is his first gastrointestinal bleed. He denies any abdominal pain.

On physical examination you find a pale, anxious, and diaphoretic elderly man with a pulse (P) of 120 and a blood pressure (BP) of 100/70 mm Hg. How do you proceed?

Continued Part B, page 284.

Name Five Causes of GI Bleed

ANSWER

1. Bleeding gastric or duodenal ulcer
2. Neoplasm: gastric, small bowel, or colonic
3. Arteriovenous malformation
4. Intussusception
5. Inflammatory bowel disease

TWO PATIENTS WITH ACUTE CHEST SYMPTOMS

You are called as the medical consultant to see **Ivan Picot,** a 42-year-old man who is recovering from cerebral aneurysm surgery, because of the acute onset of rapid respiratory rate. On physical examination, you find him to be apprehensive and acutely short of breath with a respiratory rate of 46. His BP is 130 over 80. His cardiac rate is 100. You obtain arterial blood gases, which show a pH of 7.57, Pco_2 22 mm Hg, and Po_2 65 mm Hg. He is afebrile. What diagnosis are you considering? How would you evaluate Mr. Picot?

Continued Part B, page 285.

Nicky Arachis, age two, had been coughing all night. You see him in clinic. His mother says he had a coughing spell yesterday afternoon following a quarrel over a bag of peanuts, during which he was knocked down by his older brother. He is afebrile, and physical examination of his chest is normal. What will you do?

Continued Part B, page 285.

TWO PATIENTS FROM THE ROAD

Bruce Davis, an athletic 18 year old, was quite delighted with the arrival of a new mountain bike, a graduation present from his parents. It was fitted with an aluminum frame, cantilever brakes, and 21-speed shifting. His grandparents had supplied a variety of accessories including a helmet, gel gloves, water bottles, and an antitheft lock. Unfortunately for Mr. Davis, on his first weekend trek, disaster struck. Descending a steep decline he skidded on a mass of wet leaves, resulting in a crash that threw him onto his left side. His riding companions telephoned the rescue squad from a nearby pay telephone and he was delivered by ambulance to your emergency ward.

On physical examination, you find extensive abrasions on the left side of his chest and abdomen, as well as the outside of his left leg. He complains of pain in the region of his left lower chest and asks whether a rib might be broken. On palpation, you detect left upper quadrant tenderness as well as tenderness over left lower ribs. Guarding is present. You note a P of 120 and BP of 90/60 that decreases to 70/50 on sitting upright. After placing IV lines, starting IV fluids, and sending samples of blood for type and crossmatch for possible transfusion, you will want to expedite his diagnostic work-up. What imaging examinations would you request?

Continued Part B, page 286.

Although **Darryl Halston** had received repeated warnings from his parents and girlfriend, he refused to wear his seat belt while driving his new convertible. It was not the "macho" thing to do. Furthermore, he lived in a state where the majority had voted against mandatory seat belts. This evening, at 11:00 P.M., he paid the price for his poor judgment when he was involved in a head-on collision at an intersection. The sudden deceleration threw the right side of his chest and upper abdomen against the steering wheel and steering column. Fortunately, it was not a high-velocity collision.

Mr. Halston was taken to your emergency ward; the occupants of the other car were unharmed. On your initial examination this 22-year-old man seemed hemodynamically stable. His P was measured at 90 and BP at 130/75. There was no evidence of postural changes in the upright position. He had suffered bruises and laceration to his nose, face, and hands. A major complaint, however, is right upper quadrant pain, and you are concerned by right upper quadrant tenderness and guarding. In fact, he was hyperventilating and was somewhat agitated by the severity of his pain. The chest films are unremarkable and no rib fractures are detected. How would you evaluate his right upper quadrant pain?

Continued Part B, page 286.

THREE PATIENTS WITH ACUTE ABDOMINAL SYMPTOMS

The corporate health clinic refers **George Bend,** a 52-year-old insurance actuary, to your emergency department because of right lower abdominal pain and a low-grade fever of several hours' (he thinks) duration. On physical examination, you elicit exquisite tenderness in the right lower quadrant of his abdomen. His temperature is 101.2° F and his WBC is 18,000. What is your clinical impression? Would any imaging procedure be helpful?

Continued Part B, page 287.

Tussy Pachooka, age two, is brought to the hospital at 1:00 A.M. Her worried young parents tell you she has had diarrhea all day, her stools being at first semi-formed, then liquid, and finally nothing but bloody mucus. She is screaming and has done so at intervals for six hours. She has not vomited. The past history is of no apparent relevance. She is afebrile. Peristalsis is hyperactive. Palpation reveals a slight fullness on the right side of the abdomen but no rigidity. The abdomen is soft and neither distended nor tympanitic. What are the diagnostic possibilities? Has radiology anything to offer this patient that would help narrow the differential?

Continued Part B, page 290.

Don Levine, a previously healthy 72-year-old man, was brought to your emergency department with sudden onset of severe lower abdominal and back pain, increasing in severity over the past two hours. You palpate a pulsatile abdominal mass. What is your impression? How will you evaluate this patient?

Continued Part B, page 288.

FOUR HYPERTENSIVE PATIENTS

Ronald Brewster, a 40-year-old financial analyst, has been seen by his family physician for about two years with frequent severe headaches. He also had persistently elevated BP during this time ranging from 200/120 to 160/100. During the course of these two years, he had a CT scan of the brain that was normal. He was treated with antihypertensive medication without adequate response; therefore, he was finally referred to you for a second opinion. On physical examination, you find his BP to be 170 over 120. The only other abnormal physical finding you identify is a bruit over the left abdomen. What do you think is the origin of the left abdominal bruit? Do you think it is related to his high BP? How would you evaluate him?

Continued Part B, page 291.

Priscilla Lazardi, a 41-year-old homemaker, is referred to you because of hypertension. She has a headache in association with some strenuous work such as bringing up the laundry from the basement or carrying in the groceries. Approximately a year earlier she was in an automobile accident and at the time had had three or four days of severe headache and hypertension in spite of an entirely normal computed tomogram of the brain. On physical examination, her BP is 210 over 130. She tells you that she has had medication for her high blood pressure; however, it has never really been under control. In addition to the hypertension, she also has tachycardia of about 110. What do you think is the etiology of her hypertension?

Continued Part B, page 292.

Adalena Cardoza, age 35, is admitted from clinic to your service because of abdominal pain for five days. She has been in this country only a month and a half. She tells you she has had several attacks of urinary tract infection and has passed four stones in the past 12 years. She is febrile (T 37° C), and stat urinalysis shows the presence of many WBCs and a few red blood cells (RBCs). What studies will you plan for her initially?

Continued Part B, page 291.

Mary Pastone, 72, complains of pain in her lower back increasing gradually over two years. She keeps house for her widowed son and his two children. She can recall no particular trauma to her back but is certain it always hurts more on Fridays when she carries in bags of groceries for the weekend. What film studies are in order?

Continued Part B, page 292.

FOUR PATIENTS WITH NEUROLOGICAL SYMPTOMS

Sarah Cotter, a 34-year-old economist and mother of two, underwent her first root canal filling two weeks ago; this was an experience she would like to forget. This morning she is brought to your emergency ward by her anxious husband, after she awoke with left arm and hand weakness. On further questioning you learn that Sarah is also suffering from a slowly progressive headache that began four days ago and is almost unbearable this morning. You note a fever of 100° F. Her physical examination reveals left-arm pronator drift and diminished left-hand fine finger movements. You detect weakness in her left arm muscles, especially the extensors of the wrist. The reflexes in the left arm are increased. As you start to auscultate her chest she informs you that you may hear a murmur; she has been told that she has a small atrial septal defect. What is your diagnosis? What imaging examination would you recommend in this patient?

Continued Part B, page 293.

Karen Weston, a 35-year-old stockbroker, is brought to your office by her boyfriend, who has noted several episodes of aphasia lasting five to eight minutes during the past few days. Ms. Weston is otherwise completely healthy, and her physical examination, including careful neurologic examination, is entirely normal. Do you wish to perform any imaging procedures on this patient?

Continued Part B, page 293.

Philip O'Leary, a 53-year-old roofer, specializes in custom slate work. You have been following him for over a decade, when a malignant melanoma was removed from the base of his neck. This was not a surprising diagnosis at that time, considering the excessive sunlight exposure he had received in his work. Mr. O'Leary has done well for the past ten years, although six months ago he had a local recurrence of the melanoma that was treated with additional surgery.

This afternoon, he is brought to your office by his wife, who has been observing a progressive personality change during the past six weeks, characterized by depression and forgetfulness. His co-workers have observed difficulty with his calculations and his interpretation of building plans. On physical examination, you note papilledema and difficulty with memory testing. In fact, he cannot even name the last two presidents of the United States. You also detect a mild left hemiparesis. What are your thoughts? Which imaging procedure would you recommend?

Continued Part B, page 293.

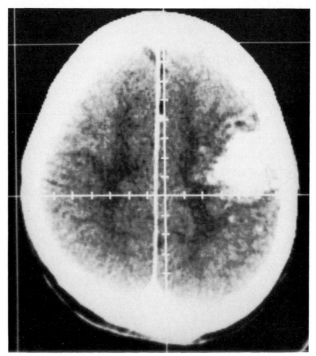

Figure 4–14 Chad Gregory, CT scan.

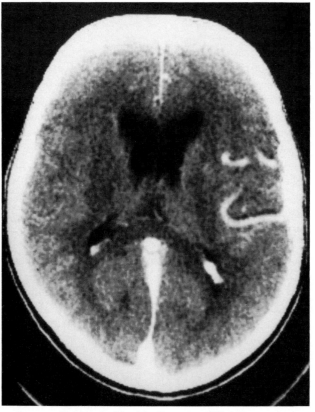

Figure 4–16 Mr. Gregory, CT scan.

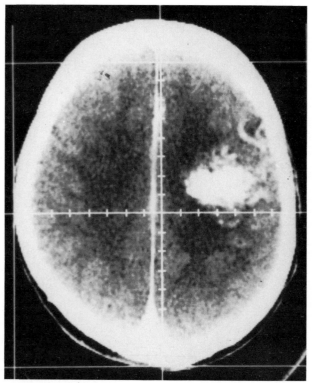

Figure 4–15 Mr. Gregory, CT scan.

Chad Gregory, a 27-year-old sailboard instructor, has noted intermittent numbness in the right side of his face and in his right arm over a six-month period, which he tried to ignore. This afternoon he is brought to your emergency ward by two companions after suffering a seizure at the shore. You learn that the seizure activity started in the right arm and progressed to a generalized seizure lasting approximately one minute. After the seizure, Mr. Gregory experienced a temporary speech impairment and a right hemiparesis lasting approximately ten minutes. Your physical examination reveals right-arm and right-facial weakness, but no papilledema. The right-arm reflexes are increased. No other abnormal physical findings are detected. You request an emergency CT scan. Figures 4–14 to 4–16 are three images from the contrast scan. What are your thoughts?

Continued Part B, page 293.

THREE SMOKERS

Paul Robertson, a 68-year-old ice cream truck vendor, comes to you with a two-and-one-half-week history of face and arm swelling as well as dyspnea on exertion. He says he has had a chronic cough for ten years. He has smoked two packs of cigarettes a day since his freshman year in high school. On physical examination, you note an elderly man with a red swollen face, swollen right arm, and distant heart sounds. The lab data included an Hb of 16 g consistent with your impression of chronic lung disease. What diagnosis are you considering to account for his facial and arm symptoms? How would you evaluate this patient?

Continued Part B, page 294.

Joe Bianti, a 52-year-old smoker and boxing promoter, was referred to you because of progressive dysphagia over several weeks. The night prior to admission he was only able to swallow liquids for dinner. He has lost over ten pounds. What are you suspecting? What examination would you request?

Continued Part B, page 294.

Denise Morton, a 47-year-old certified public accountant (CPA) and single parent, has noted an unusually severe cough, wheezing, and some shortness of breath for over two weeks. She saw blood in the coughed-up material. Denise started smoking in high school and has continued to smoke two to three packs per day since that time. Smoking has always "relaxed" her.

On physical examination, you observe a thin, tall woman with yellow-stained right index and middle fingers and clubbing. On chest auscultation, you note significant wheezing in the upper portion of the left lung. She indicates an area of tenderness in the left buttock that, on palpation, you find to be a tender, indurated, nonmovable subcutaneous mass. What do you think? How would you evaluate Mrs. Morton?

Continued Part B, page 295.

SWIM COACH WITH KNEE PAIN

Barbara Crane, a 20-year-old swimming coach, comes to your emergency department because of the acute onset of right knee pain while walking. She has no history of trauma. On physical examination, you find an exquisitely tender proximal tibia and decreased knee flexion. No effusion is detected. What are the possible diagnostic considerations? How will you work this patient up?

Continued Part B, page 299.

WOMAN WITH A BREAST MASS

Abby Xavier, a 39-year-old mother of two and district attorney, comes to you fearful that she has felt a nodule in her right breast. You confirm her impression of the palpable mass in the right breast that is located superficially near the skin surface in the upper quadrant of the breast with dimpling. The rest of her physical examination is unremarkable, including the axillary, supraclavicular, and abdominal examination. Would a mammogram be useful?

Continued Part B, page 300.

MAN WITH A TESTICULAR MASS

Jose Garcia, a 25-year-old minor-league baseball player, comes to you with a complaint of a heavy sensation in the right testis for approximately two weeks. He denies any history of trauma. On physical examination, you find a minimally tender firm right testicular mass. What diagnoses are you considering? How will you work up this patient? What imaging procedure would you request?

Continued Part B, page 301.

Question

When faced with a diagnostic problem anywhere in the body, how can you categorize possible pathologic conditions?

Answer

When faced with a diagnostic problem, think about disease categories:

Congenital
Infectious, inflammatory
Neoplastic
Thromboembolic
Other

Part B

TWO PATIENTS WITH FLU SYMPTOMS (Continued from Part A, page 260)

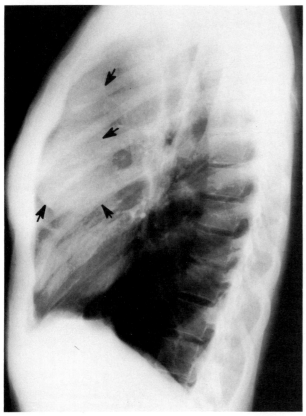

Figure 4–18 Amy Long, lateral chest radiograph.

Amy Long: *(Continued from page 260)* Adenopathy, splenomegaly, and elevated temperature imply a systemic process, such as infection or neoplasm. Infectious mononucleosis comes to mind, as well as tuberculosis, histoplasmosis, lymphoma, or Hodgkin's disease. You do a mono spot test immediately, which you find to be negative.

The chest films show a markedly widened superior mediastinum suggestive of lymphadenopathy or multiple masses. Notice that there are no pleural effusions or lung parenchymal opacities. The lateral view shows opacification of the anterior clear space confirming an anterior retrosternal location of these masses (arrows, Fig. 4–18). What do you do next? What would be the best method of diagnosing her problem?

Continued Part C, page 302.

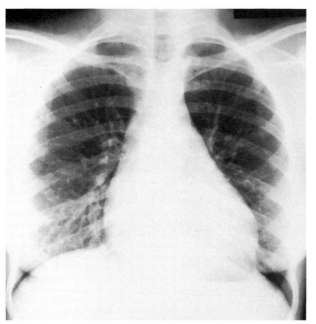

Figure 4–19 Juliana Clementine, earlier chest radiograph.

Juliana Clementine: *(Continued from page 260)* Luckily, it is apparent when submitting Ms. Clementine's name to your clerical staff that she had a chest radiograph at your institution a year earlier (Fig. 4–19). Additionally, you pick up on physical examination diminished heart sounds and a temperature of 100°F. You find on the current chest film, when compared with the previous one, a marked discrepancy in heart size, with a much larger heart size on the present examination. In view of your physical findings and the flu-like symptoms, you suspect a probable diagnosis of pericardial effusion. Such a large heart due to an acquired etiology rather than to congenital causes in the absence of congestive heart failure is usually caused either by a pericardial effusion or cardiomyopathy. How would you differentiate the two? What causes would you consider for Ms. Clementine's pericardial effusion?

Continued Part C, page 303.

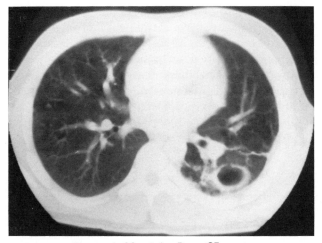

Figure 4–20 John Doe, CT scan.

Mr. Doe: *(Continued from page 261)* Figure 4–4 is the PA chest roentgenogram. On the right side, the horizontal fissure you note to be slightly higher than you expected. Eventually, Mr. Doe remembers a childhood lung infection from which he almost died, and perhaps this elevation of the horizontal fissure may be related to that illness. In the superior segment of the left lower lobe, a relatively irregular, thick-walled cavitary opacity is present (arrows on Figure 4–5, lateral view). Note its appearance on the accompanying CT scan (Fig. 4–20), which you have requested after seeing his chest films.

You might consider an abscess cavity in this alcoholic drug user. On questioning he says he has smoked for many years, and therefore you also have to consider a cavitary neoplasm. Cavitary tuberculosis is the other diagnostic consideration. Cavitary neoplasms or cavitary lesions peripheral to an intrabronchial neoplasm may occur anywhere but are more common in the upper lobes. The incidence of lung abscess from aspiration tends to be in the superior segments of the lower lobes. Tuberculous cavities are most commonly seen in the apical and posterior segments of both upper lobes, followed by the superior segment of the lower lobes. This last location is most common in women and diabetics.

Tuberculosis has a wide variety of presentations in the chest. Primary tuberculosis often (but by no means exclusively) occurs in children. Usually, the radiographic findings are not different from bacterial pneumonia unless mediastinal adenopathy accompanies the pneumonia. Most likely, the right-sided finding in Mr. Doe is due to primary tuberculous pneumonia. The tubercle bacilli are disseminated hematogenously and for a variety of reasons may take hold in various organs, for instance the lungs, kidneys, adrenals, or bone. Once disseminated, the tuberculous organisms may cause a chronic indolent infectious process in these distant organs, or the process may become dormant without any clinical manifestations. It is believed that involved dormant lymph nodes that drain the initial primary tubercular site may harbor the tuberculous organisms in an untreated patient, and for various reasons, such as stress, surgery, alcoholism, malnutrition, or drug usage, reactivation may occur leading to cavitary tuberculosis. Most likely, Mr. Doe's reactivated disease is due to drug usage and malnutrition. How would you confirm the diagnosis on Mr. Doe?

Continued Part C, page 303.

Brian Seldinger: *(Continued from page 261)* At first glance, the film looks almost normal, but considering his youth and lack of smoking history, there are probably too many interstitial markings. No old films are available for comparison. In the meantime, you obtain an arterial P_{O_2} and are somewhat surprised to find it to be only 75. No definite air bronchograms, consolidation, or atelectasis is evident. In view of the clinical presentation and minimal chest film abnormalities, what diagnoses are you entertaining?

Continued Part C, page 304.

Jeff Stitson: *(Continued from page 262)* To the amazement of both of you, a large cavitary mass is present in Jeff's left upper lobe, located in the apical posterior segment with an air-fluid level, and a small left pleural effusion is present (see Figs. 4–6 and 4–7, arrows). In spite of his vehement protests, you admit him to your service in medicine for treatment. The radiographic appearance of this cavitary density is consistent with either a tuberculous cavity or a cavitary neoplasm, but the clinical history is not consistent with either. With a tuberculous cavity the history would be much longer—weeks or months perhaps, and the symptoms much less acute.

Although neoplasm cannot be totally excluded from the history, you have never seen him smoking and lung neoplasm in a young nonsmoker would be a very unlikely diagnosis. This cavitary mass must represent an abscess cavity. Jeff gives no history of previous illness or any medical condition. Abscess may be secondary to aspiration, but more commonly, then, it would occur in the lower lobes. Numerous organisms identified on stains of the coughed-up sputum suggest a lung abscess. After extensive discussions with infectious disease and pulmonary consultants, your chief decides to order a CT scan of Jeff's chest to define the extent of the chest abnormality.

Continued Part C, page 305.

PATIENT WITH SOB (Continued from Part A, page 263)

Paul O'Grady: *(Continued from page 263)* Figure 4–8, his PA chest film, demonstrates multiple bilateral nodular densities ranging in size from 1 to 2 cm. No cardiomegaly or pleural effusions are present. Adenopathy is difficult to exclude because the nodules in the lung fields obscure the hilar and mediastinal contours. How would you evaluate the hila and mediastinum in this patient?

Continued Part C, page 305.

PATIENT WITH ACUTE BACK PAIN (Continued from Part A, page 263)

Matilda Mason: *(Continued from page 263)* PA view of the chest shows a tortuous aorta and a small left pleural effusion (Fig. 4–9). You remember seeing a relatively recent surgical scar in the right abdomen on Mrs. Mason and therefore you are quite certain that she must have a previous chest film. She tells you about her surgery approximately two months earlier for cancer in the right side of the colon. You have her husband procure the preoperative chest radiographs from a nearby hospital (Fig. 4–21). What do you think?

Continued Part C, page 305.

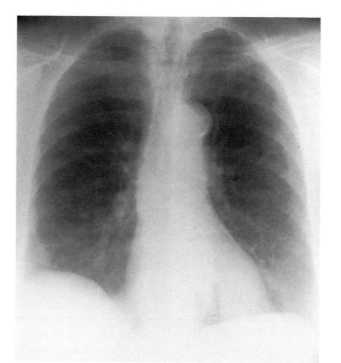

Figure 4–21 Matilda Mason, earlier PA chest radiograph.

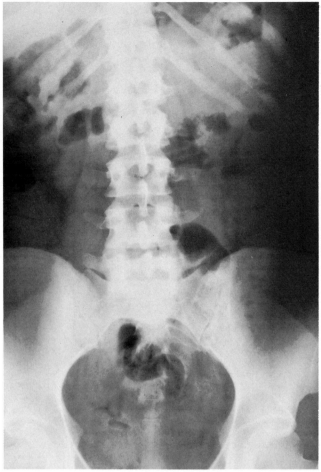

Figure 4–22 Lisa Morgan, abdominal radiograph.

Lisa Morgan: *(Continued from page 264)* Your initial request is for a supine film of the abdomen (Fig. 4–22). The soft tissue landmarks seem normal. Nothing is seen in the right lower quadrant . . . or is there? There is no intra-abdominal calcification to suggest an appendolith. Recurrent appendicitis is still a possibility, though, because only about 10 per cent of patients with acute appendicitis show a calcified appendiceal fecalith on x-ray.

What about the pattern and distribution of intestinal gas? There is a loop of mildly dilated small bowel in the midabdomen. And what about the right lower quadrant? Look again. Is there something there, or is your eye pulled back to that region because there is nothing there?

Continued Part C, page 306.

John Gaunt: *(Continued from page 264)* Had the radiologist carried out a barium enema, your patient might have suffered a severe complication, such as perforation of the colon. It is most unlikely, however, that the radiologist would have accepted a request for the enema after seeing the plain film, even if you had failed to give him the clinical history, because the film is characteristic of toxic dilatation of the colon. A barium enema is contraindicated in the face of that diagnosis (see Fig. 4–10).

Toxic dilatation is one of the most dreaded complications of ulcerative colitis—and it may occur at any time during the course of chronic disease, or it may represent the initial episode in an acute, fulminating case. Because of its anterior position as the patient lies supine, the transverse segment of the totally atonic colon shows the most striking dilatation. A careful look at the film will show the nodular protrusions of hyperplastic mucosa into the air-filled lumen of the transverse colon. The colon in this ominous condition is markedly dilated, very

thin, diffusely ulcerated, and hemorrhagic, and may show areas of actual necrosis. Since the diagnosis can be made from the history, the clinical findings, and the plain film of the abdomen, a barium enema is not only unnecessary but may well perforate this extensively diseased, thin-walled colon, causing overwhelming peritonitis.

As a matter of fact, look at the film again. Did you notice that Mr. Gaunt's colon was *already* perforated even at the time this film was made? The general radiolucency above the transverse colon, particularly in the region of the hepatic flexure and surrounding the stomach, represents free intraperitoneal air. Had an enema been done, the barium would have poured into the peritoneal cavity and added still further contamination to that already caused by spillage of blood and stool. An emergency total colectomy was performed.

End of Case

B-281

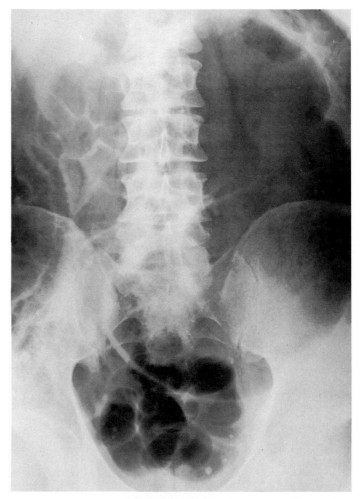

Pierre Claude: *(Continued from page 265)* You send the patient to radiology for routine chest films (negative) and for supine and upright films of the abdomen. Here is the supine film (Fig. 4–23). What and whither?

Continued Part C, page 306.

Figure 4–23 Pierre Claude, supine abdominal film.

THREE PATIENTS WITH RUQ PAIN (Continued from Part A, page 265)

Agnes Delarenzo: *(Continued from page 265)* You should have noted an elevated right hemidiaphragm, but did you see the collection of air in the liver both on the PA and lateral views with an air fluid level (Figs. 4–11 and 4–12)? How did the air get into the liver? What imaging method would you use to diagnose Mrs. Delarenzo's problem?

Continued Part C, page 306.

Leo Cleveland: *(Continued from page 266)* The combination of epigastric pain, elevated amylase, and left pleural effusion should alert you to the possibility of pancreatitis. You should have requested a CT scan. A scan at the level of the lower chest, approximately the midcardiac level, shows a left pleural effusion surrounding a soft tissue density medially that is a compression atelectasis of the left lower lobe (Fig. 4–24). Figure 4–25, at the midrenal level, demonstrates an inhomogeneous large mass that is crossing the midline (arrows). This represents a markedly enlarged and inflamed pancreas typical of acute pancreatitis. Usually, episodes of acute pancreatitis are associated with acute alcoholic episodes. However, this patient has no such history.

What other causes can you think of and what additional imaging procedures may be helpful to determine the cause of this patient's pancreatitis?

Continued Part C, page 306.

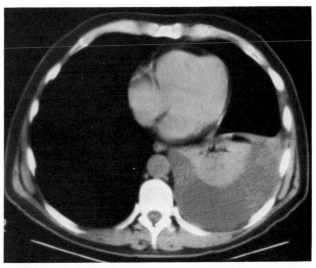

Figure 4–24 Leo Cleveland, CT scan at the midcardiac level.

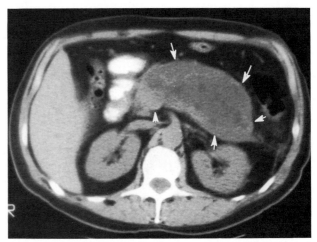

Figure 4–25 Mr. Cleveland, CT scan at the midrenal level.

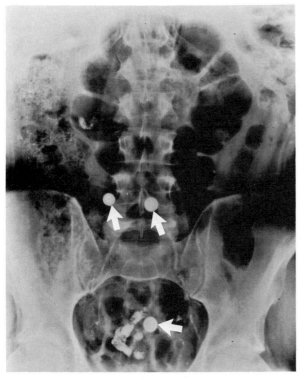

Figure 4–26 Harvey Conrad, initial abdominal film from oral cholecystogram.

Harvey Conrad: *(Continued from page 266)* This patient's history certainly suggests biliary tract disease. You order screening liver function tests and they are all normal. You order an abdominal film. Turn to Part C.

Continued Part C, page 306.

Jacques de Gautière: *(Continued from page 267)* Mr. de Gautière has obviously suffered a significant gastrointestinal bleed. Therefore he must be admitted to the hospital. A sample of blood will be sent to the blood bank for typing and cross-matching. A central venous pressure (CVP) line will be inserted to monitor fluid replacement therapy.

The most important thing to determine is whether Mr. de Gautière is *actively* bleeding now. Because the presumptive diagnosis is upper GI bleeding, most likely a duodenal ulcer in a young man of this age, a nasogastric tube is inserted and his gastric aspirate examined. If he is actively bleeding from a gastric ulcer, the gastric aspirate will be continuously bright red and will not clear with iced saline lavage. (Duodenal ulcers may or may not reflux blood into the stomach.) You do not want to do any barium studies at this point because an angiographic study for bleeding localization and therapy may be required. Most active upper GI bleeders will stop spontaneously on medical treatment without requiring emergency angiography or surgery.

Mr. de Gautière's aspirate, however, contains only specks of old blood (dark guaiac-positive material) and therefore he is probably not *actively* bleeding at this time. His barium study should be delayed until his clinical situation is stabilized for 24 to 48 hours (i.e., until his nasogastric (NG) aspirate has been monitored and found to contain no bright red blood over this period, and his vital signs and hematocrit remain stable).

Both active and inactive upper GI bleeders will benefit from fiberoptic upper endoscopy, which in most patients will localize the site of bleeding, be it in the esophagus, stomach, or duodenum. The use of *both* endoscopy and barium studies results in a definite diagnosis and visualization of the bleeding site in 98 per cent of these patients. The barium series should usually follow the endoscopy.

Now turn to page 307 and study Mr. de Gautière's upper GI series before we give you the results of the endoscopy.

Continued Part C, page 307.

Abner Lane: *(Continued from page 267)* Your immediate goal is to insert intravenous lines and administer fluids in order to begin reversing his hypotension. A blood sample is sent for stat type and crossmatching.

Did you remember to insert a nasogastric tube? In your diagnostic evaluation of this patient you must decide whether he is an upper or lower GI bleeder. Either rapidly bleeding gastritis or peptic ulcer *may* present with bright red bleeding per rectum. You do this, and the aspirate is negative for bloody material in Mr. Lane. Therefore, he is probably a lower GI bleeder. You do sigmoidoscopy to rule out bleeding hemorrhoids and other rectal sources; you find only blood coming down from above.

One hour later, with two units of blood running simultaneously as well as a liter of Ringer's lactate through a third intravenous line, his BP has risen to 105/75, but he continues to bleed per rectum. How will you locate the site of bleeding in this man's lower GI tract?

Continued Part C, page 308.

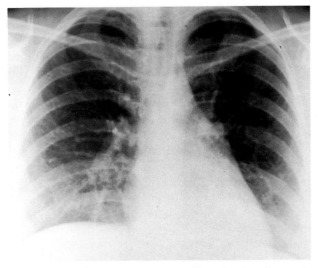

Figure 4–27 Ivan Picot, preoperative chest radiograph.

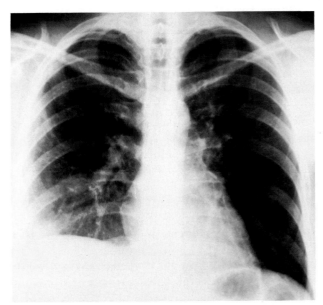

Figure 4–28 Mr. Picot, postoperative chest radiograph.

Ivan Picot: *(Continued from page 268)* You have to consider a pulmonary embolism as the most likely diagnosis, given that this patient has been immobile for several days and is in the postoperative state. Pneumonia as a cause of the symptoms is less likely in the absence of fever and cough. Because you have a preoperative chest radiograph (Fig. 4–27), it is easy for you to compare that film with the chest film that you just ordered (Fig. 4–28) and notice the difference between the two films.

Continued Part C, page 308.

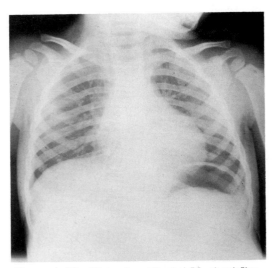

Figure 4–29 Nicky Arachis, stat PA chest film.

Nicky Arachis: *(Continued from page 268)* If you asked for a "PA chest film stat reading," you probably got a telephoned report, "normal chest," on Figure 4–29. Will you let the child go home?

Continued Part C, page 309.

PATIENTS FROM THE ROAD (Continued from Part A, page 268)

Bruce Davis: *(Continued from page 268)* He will need a stat chest film to determine whether any thoracic injuries are present. Such a film might detect a rib fracture, a pneumothorax, a pulmonary contusion, or even evidence of a ruptured left diaphragm. In searching for rib fractures, of course, a series of rib films would provide better rib detail and are frequently indicated in trauma patients. Because Mr. Davis may have suffered a serious thoracic or abdominal injury, you would not want him to stand up for his chest x-ray films as he could faint from postural hypotension and suffer further injury. Therefore, you would request the film to be taken anteroposteriorly (AP) on his stretcher. Mr. Davis' chest film is negative for signs of injury (not illustrated).

Other films you might consider taking would relate to your careful physical examination and history. In the multiple-trauma patient, these might include cervical spine series when the patient complains of neck pain, or when a multiple-trauma patient is unconscious or with altered sensorium and is unable to reliably deny the presence of neck pain. If there is a period of unconsciousness, or abnormalities on mental status on neurologic exam, a head CT scan be indicated. However, after your history and physical examination on Mr. Davis, your concern is limited to his abdomen. A likely possibility to account for his left upper quadrant pain and tenderness, as well as his tachycardia and postural hypotension, is a spleen injury with bleeding into the peritoneal cavity. Which imaging examination would you request to evaluate his abdomen?

Continued Part C, page 310.

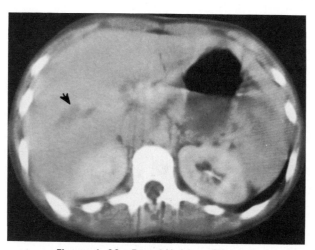

Figure 4–30 Darryl Halston, CT scan.

Darryl Halston: *(Continued from page 268)* A CT scan is in order. A slice through the right lobe of liver and both kidneys is shown in Figure 4–30. This examination was performed with intravenous contrast medium and there is faint opacification of the aorta and both kidneys and renal collecting systems. What do you think the arrow indicates?

Continued Part C, page 311.

PATIENTS WITH ACUTE ABDOMINAL SYMPTOMS
(Continued from Part A, page 269)

George Bend (*Continued from page 269*) Certainly what you are thinking about from the clinical information, examination, and lab data is appendicitis. Would you take him to surgery? That is not an unreasonable approach. However, confirmation of the clinical diagnosis can often be assisted by various imaging methods. Diagnostic ultrasound has been successfully used to identify an abnormally inflamed appendix or an appendiceal abscess. CT scanning is excellent in defining an abnormality around the appendix, as well. Go on to Part C, where you will find Mr. Bend's CT scans.

Continued Part C, page 312.

Don Levine: *(Continued from page 269)* Because the patient's vital signs are stable (BP 180/90), you immediately transfer Mr. Levine to the CT suite to rule out a leaking abdominal aortic aneurysm, which is a life-threatening condition. Figures 4–31 to 4–33 are sections through the abdomen. Figure 4–31 is at the renal level where the abdominal aorta has calcifications within its wall and appears ectatic (dilated). At the level below the kidneys you note the abdominal aorta to be markedly enlarged (Fig. 4–32). This represents an aneurysm. In the retroperitoneum, no abnormal soft tissue masses are seen to suggest leakage. Figure 4–33 is a section through the pelvis at the level of the common iliac arteries. Note the aneurysms of both common iliac arteries (arrows). Notice how close the abdominal aortic aneurysm is to the anterior abdominal wall; therefore, you can see how easy it is to palpate such a large aneurysm. Mr. Levine had a magnetic resonance (MR), and you will notice in Figure 4–34 (which is a coronal section) that it demonstrates the abdominal aortic aneurysm (with flowing blood of slightly lower signal intensity in the middle) and both common iliac artery aneurysms. A sagittal view shows the extent of this aneurysm in the anterior to posterior direction (Fig. 4–35). Although it is not always necessary, Mr. Levine did have an abdominal aortogram (Figs. 4–36 and 4–37), which showed the contrast-filled aneurysm of the aorta and iliac arteries.

At surgery, Mr. Levine had a bifurcation graft from the infrarenal aorta to the distal iliac arteries. He recovered quite nicely and uneventfully. He returned to being an enthusiastic Notre Dame football fan.

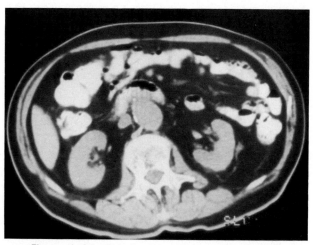

Figure 4–31 Don Levine, abdominal CT scan.

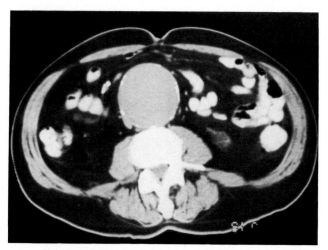

Figure 4–32 Mr. Levine, abdominal CT scan.

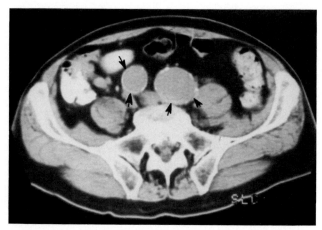

Figure 4–33 Mr. Levine, abdominopelvic CT scan.

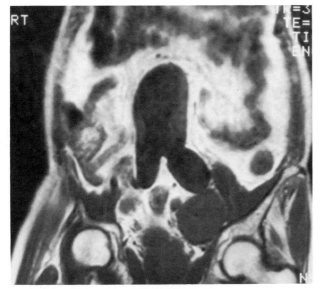

Figure 4–34 Mr. Levine, MRI scan, coronal section.

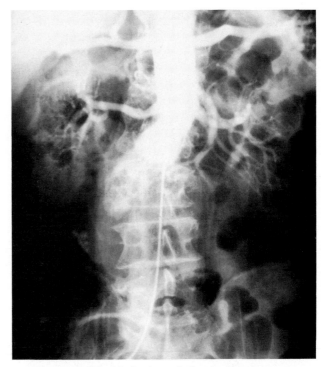

Figure 4–36 Mr. Levine, abdominal aortogram.

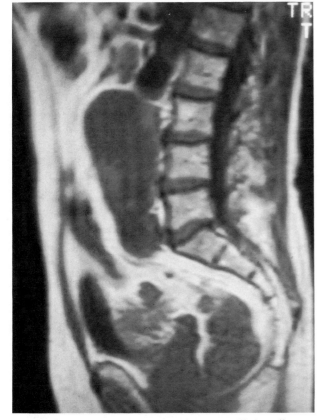

Figure 4–35 Mr. Levine, MRI scan, sagittal section.

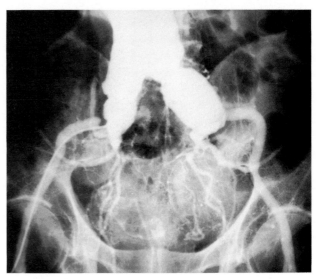

Figure 4–37 Mr. Levine, abdominal aortogram.

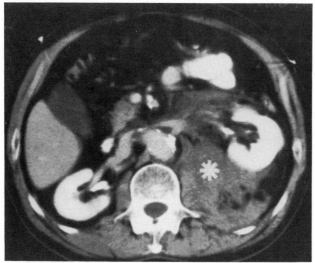

Figures 4–38 and 4–39, from a patient less fortunate than Mr. Levine who presented with a leaking abdominal aneurysm, show a sizable retroperitoneal hematoma (asterisks) that displaces the left kidney anterolaterally.

End of Case

Figure 4–38 Abdominal aortic aneurysm.

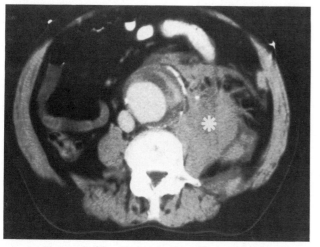

Figure 4–39 Abdominal aortic aneurysm.

Tussy Pachooka: *(Continued from page 269)* The most likely diagnosis is gastroenteritis. However, the history of bloody mucus must alert you to the possibility of an intussusception. After starting intravenous fluids you send the patient to radiology for supine and upright plain films of the abdomen. What do you think these films might show you?

Continued Part C, page 313.

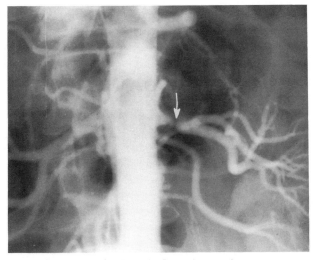

Figure 4-40 Ronald Brewster, aortogram.

Ronald Brewster: *(Continued from page 270)* The bruit in the left abdomen implies an arterial narrowing. In view of the patient's history of hypertension with a bruit, renal arterial stenosis is what you should consider even though it is actually quite rare. In order to confirm your suspicion, the appropriate study is an aortogram for visualization of the renal arteries. Figure 4-40 is his aortogram. What does it show?

The aortogram shows a marked stenosis of the proximal portion of the left renal artery (arrow). Notice the normal caliber of the right renal artery. Venous sampling has demonstrated from the left kidney elevated renin levels. How might you treat this patient?

Continued Part C, page 314.

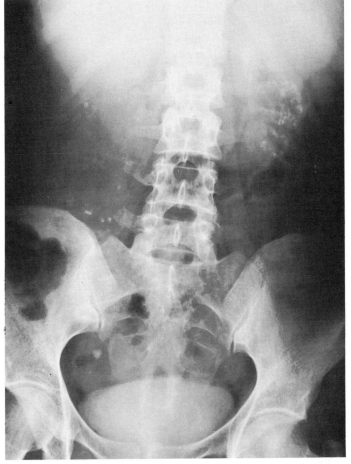

Figure 4-41 Adalena Cardoza, film from intravenous urogram.

Adalena Cardoza: *(Continued from page 270)* You will certainly have requested a plain film of her abdomen and an intravenous urogram to follow. The combination of plain abdominal film and renal ultrasound may replace intravenous urography in many clinical situations. Figure 4-41 is a 60-minute (late) film from Miss Cardoza's urogram. How would you interpret it?

Continued Part C, page 315.

Priscilla Lazardi: *(Continued from page 270)* It seems that Mrs. Lazardi has intermittent, symptomatic, severe, unresponsive hypertension. Essential hypertension, which is the most common, is more often asymptomatic and is usually not paroxysmal. It tends to respond well to antihypertensive medication. Her problem does not sound like essential hypertension. No bruit is discernible on auscultation; however, that does not totally exclude renal vascular hypertension as a cause. A pheochromocytoma causing the hypertension is a diagnosis that should enter your mind. It characteristically occurs in relatively young patients. It tends to be paroxysmal and is associated with severe symptoms. How would you evaluate Mrs. Lazardi for pheochromocytoma?

Continued Part C, page 315.

Mary Pastone: *(Continued from page 270)* Films of her lumbar spine and pelvis are certainly indicated, and here they are (Figs. 4–42 and 4–43). Do they suggest a diagnosis? What will you do next?

Continued Part C, page 315.

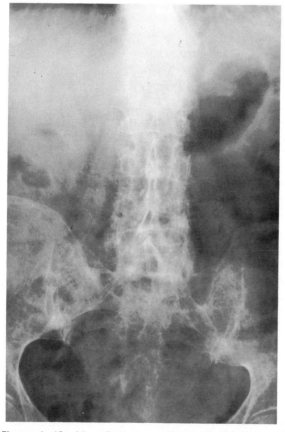

Figure 4–42 Mary Pastone, radiograph of spine and pelvis.

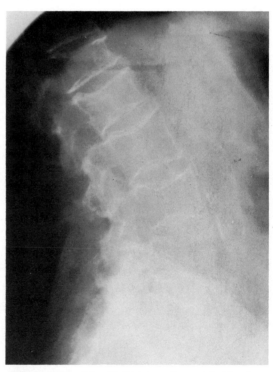

Figure 4–43 Mrs. Pastone, radiograph of spine.

Sarah Cotter: *(Continued from page 271)* Any patient presenting with the symptoms and physical findings of an acute central nervous system condition should be examined with an emergency CT scan. A variety of treatable conditions may be detected with CT, and your goal is to diagnose these as expeditiously as possible. The possibilities could include an acute bleed from a cerebral aneurysm, arteriovenous malformation, tumor, or unreported trauma. With this patient's history of a recent dental procedure and an atrial septal defect, a brain abscess is a very likely possibility. Her fever and a laboratory report of a WBC count of 22,000 further support this diagnostic possibility. What do you think of her emergency CT scan, Fig. 4–82?

Continued Part C, page 316.

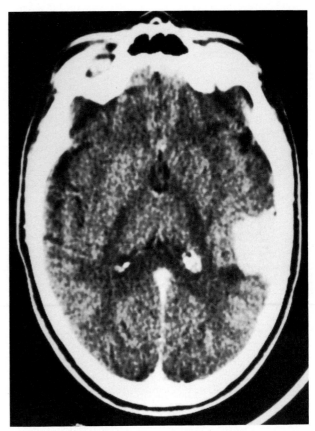

Figure 4–45 Karen Weston, CT scan.

Karen Weston: *(Continued from page 271)* Any patient presenting with such dramatic new central nervous system symptoms, even without correlative physical findings, should be examined with either CT or MRI. An image from her contrast-enhanced CT scan is shown in Figure 4–45. What do you think?

Continued Part C, page 318.

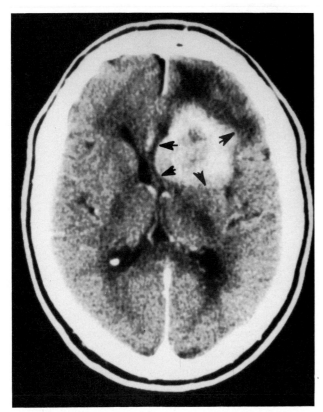

Figure 4–44 Philip O'Leary, CT scan of the brain.

Philip O'Leary: *(Continued from page 271)* Mr. O'Leary's current clinical presentation suggests a progressive central nervous system condition. You are considering the possibility of brain metastases from malignant melanoma. An image from his contrast CT scan is shown in Figure 4–44. What do you find?

Continued Part C, page 317.

Chad Gregory: *(Continued from page 272)* Assembling these three images together, you are probably visualizing a hypervascular mass in the left frontoparietal area. You are no doubt impressed by the network of curving tubular structures associated with the mass, which have the appearance of prominent blood vessels. If you thought this might be an arteriovenous malformation, you are right. Which imaging examination would confirm this diagnosis?

Continued Part C, page 318.

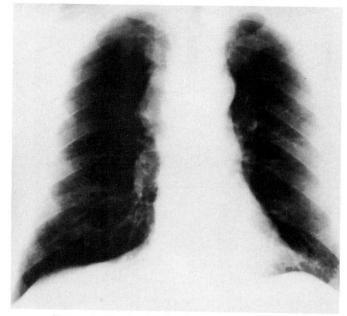

Figure 4–46 Paul Robertson, chest radiograph.

Paul Robertson: *(Continued from page 273)* Occlusion of the superior vena cava would classically present with facial rubor and swelling of upper extremities. The most common cause of superior vena caval obstruction is tumor invasion with lung cancer of lymph nodes surrounding the superior vena cava, most commonly small cell carcinoma because of its predilection for the mediastinum. Severe fibrosing mediastinitis (due to histoplasmosis, tuberculosis, or unknown etiology) may cause similar findings. You get a chest film on him (Fig. 4–46). What do you think?

Continued Part C, page 319.

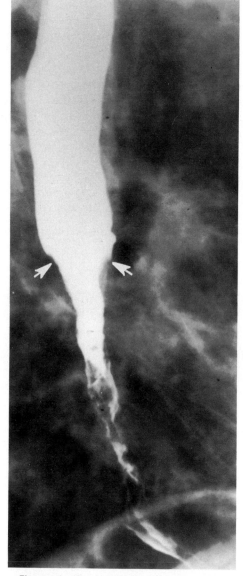

Figure 4–47 Joe Bianti, esophagram.

Joe Bianti: *(Continued from page 273)* The symptoms suggest an esophageal narrowing or obstruction, perhaps a benign stricture or a carcinoma. The weight loss usually indicates a serious problem such as an obstructing cancer and possibly distant metastases. An esophagram would be an appropriate method of examining this patient. What does the esophagram (Fig. 4–47) show? Turn to Part C for a description of the findings.

Continued Part C, page 319.

Denise Morton: *(Continued from page 273)* The most disturbing sign is Mrs. Morton's persistent wheeze, which is localized to the left upper lung. A localized wheeze always suggests a narrowing in the tracheobronchial tree. In asthmatics it is generalized, temporary, and produced by bronchoconstriction. In Mrs. Morton's case, the persistent wheeze suggests mechanical narrowing of a bronchus in the left upper lobe. A bronchogenic carcinoma is the likely diagnosis in view of her strong smoking history. Bronchial adenoma or aspirated foreign body are far less likely. You request PA and lateral chest radiographs on Mrs. Morton (Figs. 4–48 and 4–49).

Continued Part C, page 319.

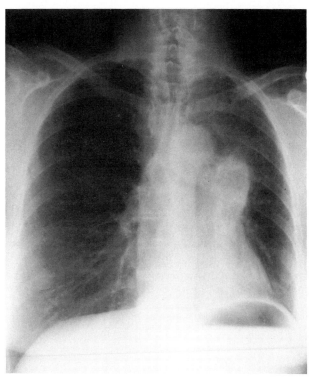

Figure 4–48 Denise Morton, PA chest radiograph.

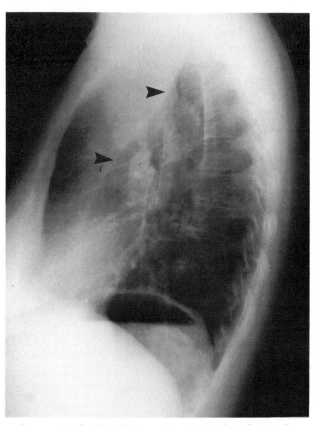

Figure 4–49 Mrs. Morton, lateral chest radiograph.

Bruce Gunzel: *(Continued from page 274)* Hematuria is a symptom associated with some abnormality of the kidneys, ureters, urinary bladder, or urethra. Usually, a calculus is associated with severe pain. A blood clot in a patient with bleeding disorder or one who is on heparin may also cause hematuria without pain. Trauma is a possible cause for hematuria. Neoplasm from the kidneys, ureter, or bladder can also cause hematuria. The elevation of the hemoglobin, which is unexpected in the presence of acute bleeding, might make you think of production of erythropoietin by a tumor, usually a renal cell carcinoma, originating from the kidney. An intravenous urogram was done first. The nephrotomogram is Figure 4–50. What do you think?

Continued Part C, page 320.

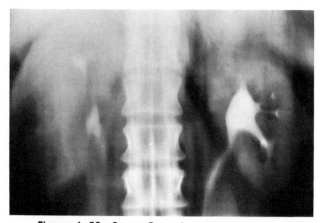

Figure 4–50 Bruce Gunzel, nephrotomogram.

Ernest Jones: *(Continued from page 274)* You would request an intravenous urogram (Fig. 4–51) because of his hematuria. His symptoms suggest bladder outlet obstruction, most frequently caused by benign prostatic hypertrophy in a man of his age.

Rectal examination is normal, however, and so you must consider other causes for Mr. Jones' symptoms. Both large bladder tumors and bladder stones may present as bladder outlet obstruction. Gross hematuria is a common symptom for both of these entities, especially when accompanied by cystitis. It should be kept in mind, however, that episodes of gross hematuria may occur with uncomplicated benign prostatic hypertrophy; dilated veins that develop at the bladder neck may rupture when the patient strains to void.

When reviewing Mr. Jones' urogram you should also be alert for signs of renal and ureteral neoplasms, calculi, and renal cysts. These conditions may produce hematuria. Did you ask for a chest film? Please turn to Part C and evaluate the films provided.

Continued Part C, page 320.

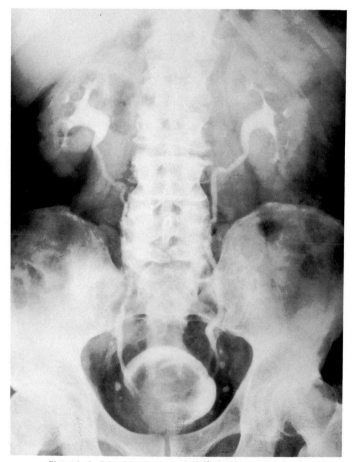

Figure 4–51 Mr. Jones, intravenous urogram.

Bertha Taylor: *(Continued from page 275)* Her low Hb and guaiac-positive stools are consistent with gastrointestinal bleeding. Her stable vital signs and slowly progressive symptoms are suggestive of a chronic or slow bleed. The potential sites of bleeding include lesions in the stomach, duodenum, the rest of the small bowel, or colon. A nasogastric aspirate shows no evidence of new or old blood—it is guaiac-negative. So you are considering a small bowel or colonic lesion. Colonic bleeding may be caused by colonic neoplasm, diverticulosis, inflammatory bowel disease, and very rarely, arteriovenous malformation. The plain film of the abdomen is normal. What examination would you request?

Continued Part C, page 321.

Adele Grabet: *(Continued from page 275)* Her history of early satiety suggests a gastric problem such as a benign ulcer or a neoplasm. Because of the significant weight loss, a neoplasm is much more likely and could also be the cause of bleeding resulting in the guaiac-positive stool. Figure 4–52 is a film from her upper GI series. The single film shows an irregularly narrowed distal antrum with masses projecting into the barium-filled lumen (arrows). The appearance suggests a gastric neoplasm, probably an adenocarcinoma of the stomach. A metastatic neoplasm is also possible such as occurs from a breast primary cancer. Following this upper GI series, Mrs. Grabet underwent endoscopy and endoscopic biopsy, which was interpreted as mucin-producing adenocarcinoma of the stomach. Superficial mucosal ulcerations were noted at endoscopy, explaining her GI bleeding. How will you stage this tumor?

Continued Part C, page 321.

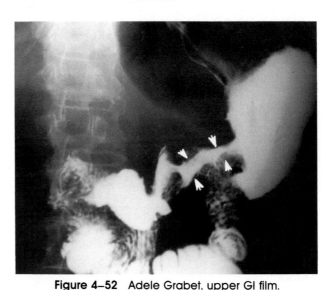

Figure 4–52 Adele Grabet, upper GI film.

Juan Rivera: *(Continued from page 275)* The most important determination is whether the jaundice is caused by mechanical obstruction of the biliary tree or by hepatocellular disease. In addition to the laboratory data of direct bilirubin (which if it is elevated is more indicative of mechanical obstruction), ultrasound examination is the quickest way to determine the presence of biliary dilatation. Look at Figures 4–53 and 4–54. Figure 4–53 is an ultrasound study of a very dilated common bile duct (between cursors). Figure 4–54 is an ultrasound study through the body of pancreas that shows a markedly dilated pancreatic duct (between markers).

Hepatitis involving the liver parenchyma could cause hepatocellular jaundice; a laboratory examination would then point to nonobstructive jaundice. A variety of conditions may cause obstructive jaundice. Calculi may occur in the gallbladder and may travel and obstruct the common bile duct and may even lodge in the ampulla. All these calculi may potentially cause obstructive jaundice. A neoplastic process arising from the pancreas (area of the head of the pancreas), the common bile duct, ampulla of

Vater, the gallbladder or the liver itself, or the porta hepatis all may cause obstructive jaundice. Metastatic neoplasms to the porta hepatis cause jaundice by extrinsic compression of the common bile duct. An inflammatory process may involve the pancreas causing acute pancreatitis that can be a cause of jaundice by obstructing the common bile duct. Acute cholecystitis and cholangitis with cholelithiasis may also cause jaundice.

If gallbladder disease seems clinically to be the most likely cause for Mr. Rivera's jaundice, ultrasound is the examination of choice. If abnormality of the pancreas, on the other hand, is more likely, then CT is the initial method of study because it will define the pancreas, the porta hepatis, and the liver more completely than ultrasound. Because this patient's jaundice was basically painless, the possibility of an abnormality of the head of the pancreas is most likely. Analyze the CT section in Figure 4–55.

Continued Part C, page 321.

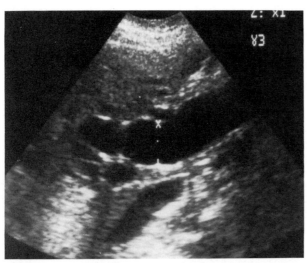

Figure 4–53 Juan Rivera, ultrasound study of the common bile duct.

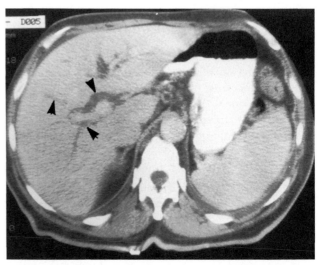

Figure 4–55 Mr. Rivera, CT scan of the pancreas.

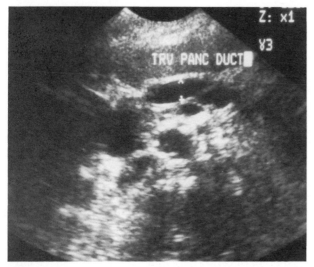

Figure 4–54 Mr. Rivera, ultrasound study through the body of the pancreas.

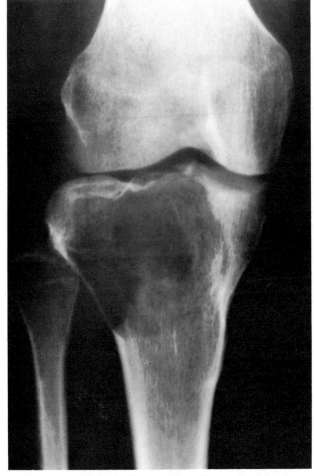

Figure 4–56 Barbara Crane, AP radiograph of the knee.

Barbara Crane: *(Continued from page 276)* Because there is no specific trauma history in this case, you should always consider the possibility of an underlying process in a patient with a new onset of bone pain. Therefore, in this patient you should consider a process such as a bone cyst or possibly a benign or malignant tumor with a pathologic fracture. In an elderly patient, osteoporosis may be the cause of a pathologic fracture. You would start the evaluation with the request for plain films of the knee (Fig. 4–56). What do you think?

Continued Part C, page 322.

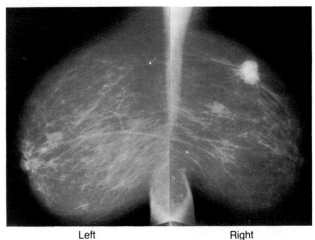

Left   Right

Figure 4–57 Abby Xavier, mammogram, lateral view.

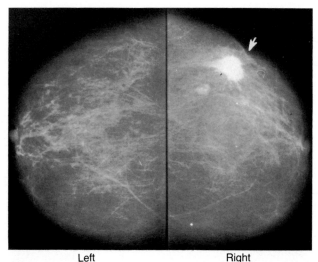

Left   Right

Figure 4–58 Mrs. Xavier, mammogram, craniocaudad view.

Abby Xavier: *(Continued from page 276)* Yes, it may help to differentiate cancer from benign lesions, such as fibroadenomas or cysts and may identify other abnormalities not palpable on physical examination. Figure 4–57 is a film screen mammogram, lateral view of both breasts that shows an irregular spiculated mass in the right upper quadrant. This radiographic appearance is highly suggestive of breast cancer. Figure 4–58 is the craniocaudad view of both breasts that localizes the spiculated mass to the outer quadrant and demonstrates skin dimpling (arrow). Whether this lesion has metastasized also is an important question. How will you determine this?

Continued Part C, page 323.

Jose Garcia: *(Continued from page 276)* A palpable testicular mass in a young man is always suspect for a neoplasm. In this case, it is the most likely diagnosis. Hematoma may be considered, although a history of trauma usually accompanies that diagnosis. Other causes of palpable scrotal masses include hydrocele and epididymitis. Testicular torsion would present with acute exquisite tenderness. You requested testicular ultrasound. Compare the echo texture of the left and right testes in Figure 4–59. What do you think?

(Answer upside down at bottom of page.)

Figure 4–59   Jose Garcia, ultrasound study.

Jose Garcia: The left testis has a normal echo pattern (open arrowheads) define the testicular borders). There is a well-defined mass with a different echo pattern within the right testis (arrows). This abnormal echo pattern is suggestive of a testicular tumor. What staging examinations would you request?

Continued Part C, page 324.

Brian Seldinger: *(Continued from page 279)* Any patient with an almost normal chest film, cough, and dypsnea without chest pain (as compared with acute pulmonary embolism, usually associated with chest pain), and especially with laboratory-proven hypoxemia, should be considered as a candidate for possible *Pneumocystis carinii* pneumonia (PCP). Therefore, you decide to pursue a history of risk factor for HIV infection.

Mr. Seldinger reports a previous episode of candida esophagitis treated about four months ago while traveling in the Caribbean. He also reports occasional homosexual encounters. With this new information, the possibility of HIV-related PCP is high on your differential. Mr. Seldinger consents to an HIV test, which is reported to be positive.

The differential diagnostic considerations include, in addition to PCP, viral pneumonia due to herpes or other viruses. In a patient who is HIV positive, bacterial pneumonia tends to be more localized or nodular, may be accompanied by pleural effusions, or may be characterized by consolidation, rather than a diffuse process, as in this case.

A neoplastic condition also has to enter the differential diagnosis in this patient and that is Kaposi's sarcoma. In general, this occurs in older homosexual male patients who often have skin manifestations of Kaposi's sarcoma. The chest radiographic findings tend to be confluent nodular densities in the mid- and lower lung zones with pleural effusions and sometimes hilar adenopathy. Adenopathy and pleural effusions are quite uncommon with PCP.

A definitive diagnosis is important for proper treatment, and therefore some specimen has to be obtained through sputum, tracheal aspirate, or possibly bronchoscopic aspiration or bronchoalveolar lavage. Mr. Seldinger had bronchoscopy with BAL (bronchoalveolar lavage), which yielded *Pneumocystis carinii.* He was treated and responded within days, and two weeks later he was back to selling bicycles.

Incidentally, acute PCP may be associated with a normal chest film in its early course. A specialized examination such as a gallium scan or a high-resolution CT scan may sometimes be helpful in this very early stage to diagnose PCP.

Figure 4–64 is a PA chest roentgenogram of a 22-year-old drug addict who presented with high fever, a heart murmur, and chest pain. What findings do you see? What is your diagnosis?

Proceed to page 326.

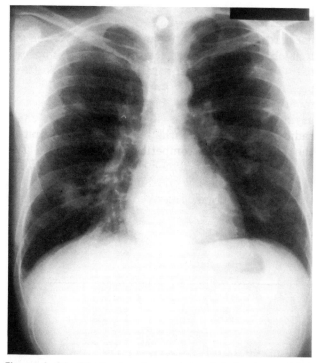

Figure 4–64   PA chest radiograph in a febrile drug addict.

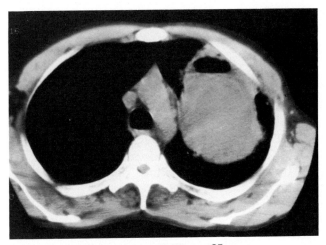

Figure 4–65   Jeff Stitson, CT scan.

Jeff Stitson: *(Continued from page 280)* Figure 4–65 is a CT scan of the chest at the level of the aortic arch that shows a large soft tissue mass with an air-fluid level consistent with an abscess cavity. No intrabronchial lesions were noted on any of the sections. Jeff was placed on antibiotics, initially intravenously, and then was switched to oral antibiotics. He recovered completely, and a chest film was normal several weeks later. In strictest confidence, he later told you that he has had a seizure disorder since childhood. Although it has usually responded well to anticonvulsive therapy, he did experience a seizure in the two weeks prior to admission and presumably aspirated at that time, at night while asleep on his back.

End of Case

PATIENT WITH SHORTNESS OF BREATH (SOB) (Continued from Part A, page 280)

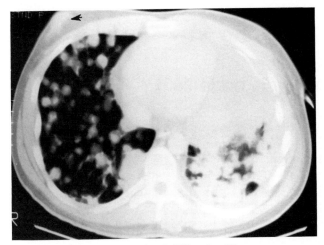

Figure 4–66   Paul O'Grady, CT scan.

Paul O'Grady: *(Continued from page 280)* You requested a CT scan, which confirms multiple pulmonary nodules (Fig. 4–66). No hilar or mediastinal adenopathy was seen on higher sections. In addition, a subcutaneous nodule (arrow) in the right chest wall is apparent. (Did you miss it?) You are, of course, considering a diagnosis of multiple pulmonary metastases. In order to treat this patient, you need to make a specific diagnosis, preferably a primary site determination. How would you determine Mr. O'Grady's primary tumor site? What type of neoplasm may spread to the lung?

Continued Part D, page 327.

PATIENT WITH ACUTE BACK PAIN (Continued from Part B, page 280)

Matilda Mason: *(Continued from page 280)* A previous PA film shows no pleural effusion on the left (Fig. 4–61), and although she has a calcified tortuous aorta on the preoperative examination, there is a significant change of the contour of the superior mediastinum with considerable irregularity and fullness on the current examination. What diagnosis are you thinking about? What diagnostic procedures can you think of to make a diagnosis?

Continued Part D, page 327.

PATIENT WITH DIARRHEA (Continued from Part B, page 264)

Lisa Morgan: *(Continued from page 264)* If you are suspicious of the overall "grayness" of the right lower quadrant and the lack of bowel gas in this area—you are right. What should you suspect? A tumor could cause this, displacing air-filled bowel away from the area. An inflammatory mass or an abscess in this region, causing irritation of the lower psoas muscle on the right and pain on hyperextension of the leg, could also account for the x-ray and physical findings. On the chance that the patient might have appendicitis, a barium enema was considered. Would you request that study on this patient?

Continued Part D, page 328.

Pierre Claude: *(Continued from page 282)* The plain film of the abdomen shows some scattered gas in small bowel loops on the right side of the abdomen. There is a huge, gas-filled structure occupying most of the left side of the abdomen. Some mottled densities within it suggest fecal material. What do you think has happened and what would you do next?

Continued Part D, page 329.

PATIENTS WITH RUQ PAIN (Continued from Part B, page 283)

Agnes Delarenzo: *(Continued from page 282)* Mrs. Delarenzo is an elderly febrile hypotensive woman with shaking chills and exquisite tenderness in the right upper abdomen. You should suspect septic shock caused by an abscess in either the liver or the gallbladder, in a subdiaphragmatic location, or possibly related to the right kidney. You would want to get a CT scan of the abdomen on Mrs. Delarenzo to define the precise location of this air-fluid-containing cavity.

Continued Part D, page 330.

Harvey Conrad: *(Continued from page 283)* The arrows point to metallic snaps on his boxer shorts (Fig. 4–26). No calcified gallstones are seen. Only 10 to 15 per cent of gallstones are sufficiently calcified to be seen on a plain film of the abdomen. Therefore an abdominal film is not necessary when you suspect gallbladder disease.

What do you do next?

Continued Part D, page 332.

Leo Cleveland: *(Continued from page 283)* Gallstone pancreatitis is the second most common cause of acute pancreatitis. It is usually caused by a common bile duct stone lodged in the duodenal ampulla of Vater that obstructs both the common bile duct and the pancreatic duct, causing the backup of the pancreatic duct and pancreatitis. Therefore, a gallbladder ultrasound would be the appropriate examination in this patient.

Continued Part D, page 331.

Jacques de Gautière: *(Continued from page 284)*
The upper GI series shows a classic acute duodenal ulcer crater with edematous mucosal folds radiating from the crater, but no deformity to suggest prior ulcer disease and scarring (Fig. 4–67). This ulcer crater is best seen on the air contrast spot films (Fig. 4–68) and cannot be seen on the stomach film, where the bulb is filled with barium (see Fig. 4–67).

The patient was started on cimetidine and antacids and made an excellent recovery. In retrospect, endoscopy was probably not necessary. It is often omitted in similar patients with no evidence of *active* bleeding on gastric lavage in this age group, since there is such a high probability that the working diagnosis will be duodenal ulcer disease.

End of Case

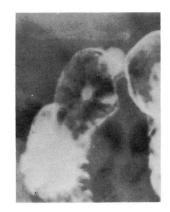

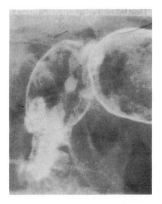

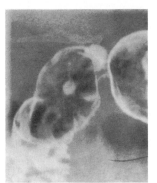

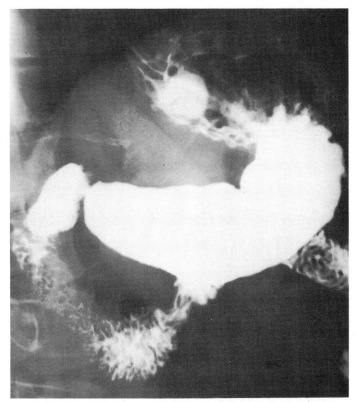

Figure 4–67 Mr. de Gautière, spot films of duodenal bulb.

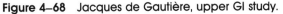

Figure 4–68 Jacques de Gautière, upper GI study.

Abner Lane: *(Continued from page 284)* An emergency barium enema on a hypotensive patient with active lower GI bleeding and an unprepared colon is usually unrewarding. It would be impossible to differentiate feces and blood clots from possible pathologic lesions within the colon. In addition, if the cause of bleeding is diverticulosis, the barium study cannot tell you which diverticulum is bleeding. Furthermore, the introduction of barium would prevent the use of angiographic localization of the bleeding site, because retained barium would obscure the field.

An attempt at colonoscopy would also probably be unrewarding, and it might also be difficult and hazardous to negotiate the scope through an unprepared and blood-filled colon. Furthermore, it might not be possible to recognize the bleeding site in the presence of so much blood. A nuclear scan may localize a bleeding site, but will not show the bleeding lesion precisely.

You refer the patient for angiography. Please turn to Part D and interpret the initial superior mesenteric arteriogram.

Continued Part D, page 333.

PATIENTS WITH ACUTE CHEST SYMPTOMS (Continued from Part B, page 285)

Ivan Picot: *(Continued from page 285)* Figure 4–27 shows normal lung fields, normal heart size, and no pleural effusions. On the examination that you just obtained on Mr. Picot there is a small patchy density in the right costophrenic angle, and the right diaphragm seems very slightly elevated (see Fig. 4–28). These findings are extremely subtle. However, the very subtle abnormality in the chest radiograph and the clinical history should make you even more suspicious of a pulmonary embolism. The subtle chest radiographic findings are consistent with pulmonary emboli. However, more definitive methods of diagnosis are necessary. What are these methods of confirmation for pulmonary embolism?

Continued Part D, page 334.

Nicky Arachis: *(Continued from page 285)* We hope not. Any child in whom inhalation of a foreign body is possible from the history should have inspiration-expiration films. The bronchus normally dilates during inspiration and narrows during expiration. When a foreign body interferes with egress of air from one lung, air will be "trapped" on the obstructed side and there may be demonstrable mediastinal shift at expiration as the nonobstructed lung empties. Any single chest film will be obtained at full inspiration (Fig. 4–69), when, indeed, the mediastinum may be in midposition. Figure 4–70 is Nicky's expiration film. Compare Figures 4–71 and 4–72 with Figures 4–68 and 4–70.

Obviously there is mediastinal shift at expiration, and there must be a (nonopaque) foreign body in the left main bronchus with air trapping behind it. A peanut *(Arachis hypogaea)* was recovered at bronchoscopy. Had you let this child go home, he might well have developed atelectasis and infection in the obstructed lobe before the correct diagnosis could be established.

End of Case

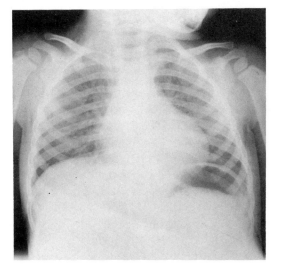

Figure 4–69 Nicky Arachis, chest radiograph at inspiration.

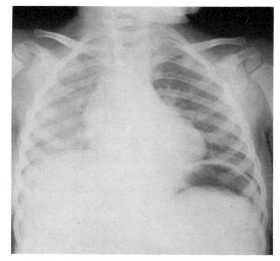

Figure 4–70 Nicky Arachis, chest radiograph at expiration.

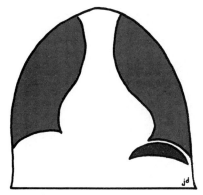

Figure 4–71 Inspiration.

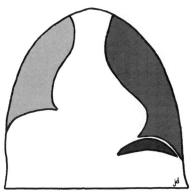

Figure 4–72 Expiration.

Bruce Davis: *(Continued from page 286)* You arrange for an emergency CT scan of the abdomen because it is a fast, accurate, and reliable technique for detecting the presence of abdominal and retroperitoneal injuries, and also for evaluating their extent.

Here are two images from his CT examination. Figure 4–73 is a slice taken through the liver and spleen. Figure 4–74 shows the lower abdomen just below the kidneys. This study was performed following an intravenous infusion of contrast medium, which has opacified the blood vessels. Note the white round aorta in Figure 4–73 and the portal venous vessels within the liver. This patient had also been given oral contrast material to opacify loops of bowel, best seen in Figure 4–74. The diagonal band of diminished x-ray attenuation (asterisk in the darker band) through the anterior portion of the spleen represents blood within a splenic fracture. Hematoma within the fracture is less dense than the opacified splenic parenchyma on either side of it. Figure 4–74 informs you that hemoperitoneum is present. The large collection of low density in the *right* flank is free blood in the peritoneal cavity. Surgery is now indicated. Note how the collection of blood (black asterisk) lying between the psoas muscle (P) and the abdominal wall muscles (arrows) displaces the right colon (white asterisk) medially and anteriorly. At laparotomy, the lacerated spleen could not be repaired and splenectomy was performed. His postoperative course was most satisfactory.

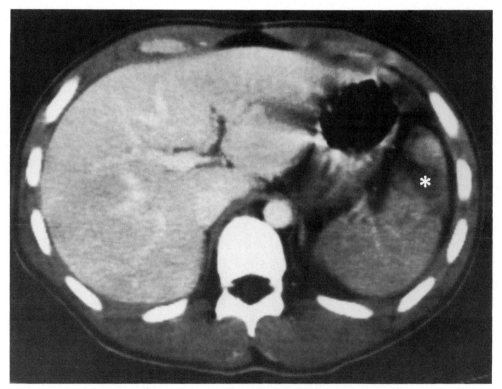

Figure 4–73 Bruce Davis, CT scan of liver and spleen.

Although you might have considered requesting plain films of the abdomen, in this patient they would not have been helpful in identification of an abdominal organ injury and would have delayed CT scanning. An immediate plain chest film is always indicated in the multiple-trauma patient because a variety of thoracic injuries usually detectable on the film, such as pneumothorax, may be quickly identified and treated. You may have considered diagnostic peritoneal lavage instead of CT to detect hemoperitoneum; however, much more information is provided by CT if the patient is sufficiently stable to travel to the CT scanner for 30 minutes. Peritoneal lavage, performed in the emergency department, would be the examination of choice in the *unstable* patient who could not be moved to the CT facility.

End of Case

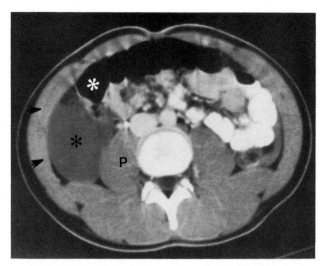

Figure 4-74 Mr. Davis, CT scan of lower abdomen.

Darryl Halston: *(Continued from page 286)* The irregular low-density area indicated by the arrow represents a liver laceration. The lower attenuation blood within the laceration appears darker than the contrast-opacified normal liver parenchyma. The CT scan is somewhat suboptimal in quality because of hyperventilation related to his level of pain and anxiety. The streak artifacts radiating from the stomach are a combination of motion and changes in CT attenuation related to the fluid level of beer in his stomach. The remainder of the CT scan (not shown) was unremarkable, showing no evidence of free blood in the peritoneal cavity (hemoperitoneum). Do you think this patient will need surgery or can he be managed conservatively?

Continued Part D, page 334.

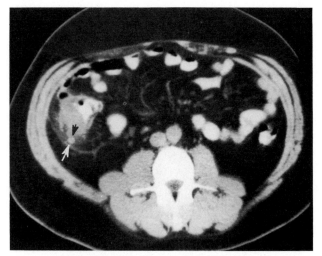

Figure 4–75 George Bend, CT scan.

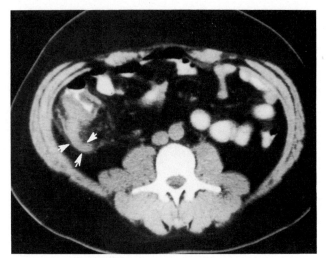

Figure 4–76 Mr. Bend, CT scan.

George Bend: *(Continued from page 287)* CT is the correct imaging procedure. Figures 4–75 and 4–76 are CT scans at the level of the appendix and cecum. Figure 4–75 shows a soft tissue mass at the tip of the cecum that is displacing the contrast within the cecum itself. Some pericecal fatty infiltrations are suggestive of an inflammatory process. In addition, there is a tiny opacity that represents an appendolith (arrows). Figure 4–76 shows the enlarged irregular appendix (arrows) with periappendiceal fat infiltration and a soft tissue mass in the tip of the cecum that represents the appendiceal abscess.

Because of the other differential diagnostic considerations such as mesenteric adenitis, viral syndrome, and perhaps even Crohn's disease, the specific demonstration of an inflamed appendix and an appendiceal abscess is important. Mr. Bend was treated with antibiotics and several days later had an appendectomy and made an uneventful recovery.

Figure 4–77 is another patient with acute appendicitis in whom an ultrasound examination shows a thickened, sausage-shaped appendix (arrows) in the longitudinal projection. The asterisk shows periappendiceal fluid. Figure 4–78 shows the thick edematous appendix on cross section (arrows). At ultrasound, a normal appendix is most often not visualized.

End of Case

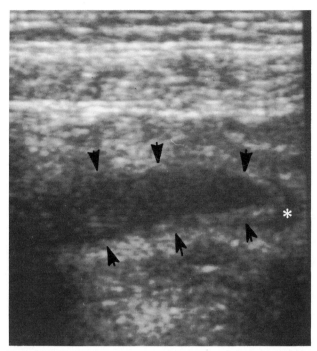

Figure 4–77   Acute appendicitis, ultrasound study (longitudinal).

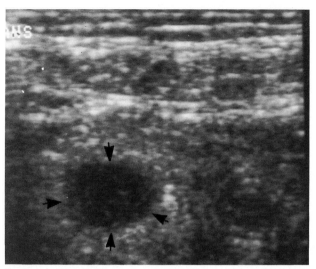

Figure 4–78   Acute appendicitis, ultrasound study (transverse).

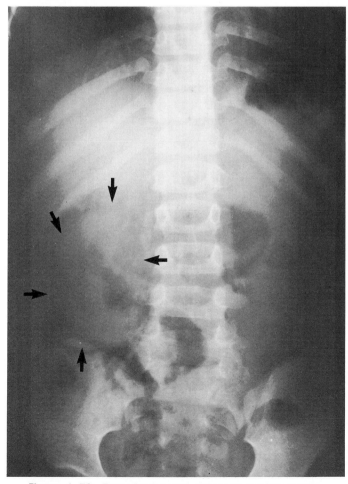

Figure 4–79   Tussy Pachooka, abdominal radiograph.

Tussy Pachooka: *(Continued from page 290)* The erect film showed no free air or abnormal fluid levels. Here is the supine plain film (Fig. 4–79). Does it help you?

Yes, there *is* a round soft tissue mass on the right side of the abdomen between the twelfth rib and the iliac crest. The scattered gas shadows tell you nothing except that there is no roentgen evidence of intestinal obstruction. The presence of a mass with her history is very suggestive of intussusception, usually ileocolic in a young child. What will you do next?

Continued Part D, page 336.

Ronald Brewster: *(Continued from page 291)* A relatively new method of treatment for a stenotic artery is dilatation by the radiologist with a special balloon catheter, a so-called angioplasty. In fact, Mr. Brewster had left renal arterial angioplasty, and Figure 4–80 shows the normal caliber of the left renal artery after the procedure. BP came down within the next two hours to a normal level of approximately 120 over 60.

Mr. Brewster had a simple straightforward presentation of hypertension and an important physical finding of a bruit suggesting the etiology to be renal vascular. Even though, in virtually every patient, this renal arterial stenosis is a possible cause of hypertension, much more frequently the etiology is unknown and the hypertension is idiopathic. When the physical finding of a bruit is not present, a much more involved work-up is necessary. A renal ultrasound may be an initial work-up to identify asymmetry in the size of the kidneys. A small kidney might indicate long-standing ischemia due to renal arterial stenosis. Symmetrical size of both kidneys would be against renal vascular etiology of hypertension. A renal scan "nuclear" study can assess renal blood flow. Asymmetry of blood flow to one of the kidneys is highly suggestive of a vascular etiology for hypertension. A captopril test can suggest a vascular etiology for the hypertension. A "hypertensive intravenous urogram" was used in the past, but at this time it is only of historic interest and should not be the method of evaluation for hypertensive patients.

End of Case

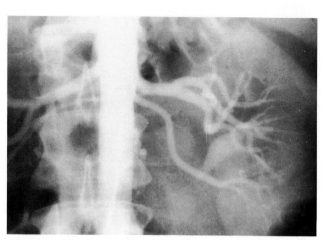

FIGURE 4–80 Ronald Brewster, after renal arterial angioplasty.

Adalena Cardoza: *(Continued from page 291)* The urogram shows numerous calcifications, apparently located in the kidneys. A detail film shows blunted and crowded calices and loss of cortex, indicating pyelonephritis in that kidney (Fig. 4–81). At the same time the laboratory results show an elevated serum calcium (12.5) and a decrease in serum phosphorus (2.1). What next?

Continued Part D, page 337.

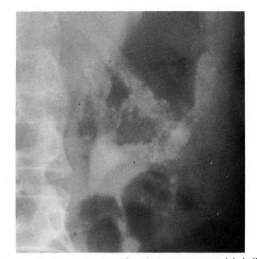

Figure 4–81 Adalena Cardoza, urogram (detail).

Priscilla Lazardi: *(Continued from page 292)* The clinical test is 24-hour urine for vanillylmandelic acid (VMA) and metanephrins. In Mrs. Lazardi, both were markedly elevated indicating pheochromocytoma. How would you locate the pheochromocytoma?

Continued Part D, page 338.

Mary Pastone: *(Continued from page 292)* Films of the spine certainly show pronounced bone loss. Note that in the lateral view the density of the vertebral bodies is not much greater than that of the soft tissues anterior to them. The intervertebral discs seem to be expanding at the expense of the bony end-plates of the bodies of the vertebrae. No lytic areas are seen, but one lumber vertebra looks collapsed. (Calcification is noted within a widened abdominal aorta.) You make a presumptive diagnosis of osteoporosis.

Two weeks later, Mrs. Pastone returns to the emergency room with a fracture of the humerus near the elbow, which occurred spontaneously when she lifted a heavy frying pan. With this history and with the discovery of anemia, you decide to admit her for study.

What will you request?

Continued Part D, page 338.

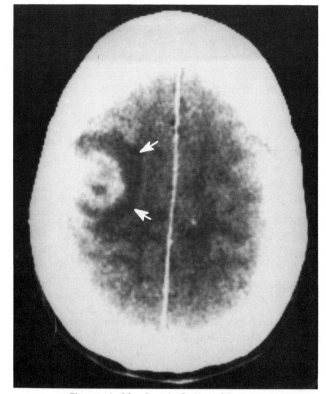

Figure 4–82   Sarah Cotter, CT scan.

Sarah Cotter: *(Continued from page 293)* Figure 4–82 (contrast scan) shows marked inhomogeneous enhancement in a right frontal mass, which appears to have a small low-attenuation center. The surrounding edema is hypodense around the enhancing lesion (arrows). Note how well the falx cerebri (midline vertical white line) is also enhanced with intravenous contrast material because of the contrast enhancement of the falx blood vessels.

The mass is characteristic in appearance for a brain abscess with a necrotic center and surrounding edema. Although a contrast-enhancing brain tumor may also appear similar, this patient's clinical history and the thick rind of surrounding edema suggest brain abscess as a more likely possibility. Figure 4–83 is an MR scan (T2-weighted image) that was also requested; the mass has an increased MR signal in an inhomogeneous pattern. The central lower signal area probably represents cystic necrosis within the abscess.

Mrs. Cotter was scheduled for an emergency craniotomy. Needle aspiration of the mass revealed pus. She was treated with abscess drainage and intravenous antibiotics. Cultures of the abscess grew streptococcus. Although prophylactic antibiotics may diminish the likelihood of systemic infection in patients with intracardiac left-to-right shunts during dental procedures, they may not eliminate them entirely. Moreover, one should consider the possibility of an acute brain abscess in a patient such as Sarah Cotter, especially when the clinical presentation makes this diagnosis so likely.

End of Case

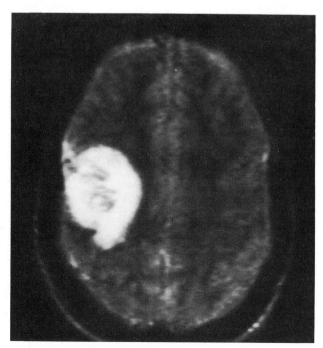

Figure 4–83   Mrs. Cotter, MRI scan.

Philip O'Leary: *(Continued from page 293)* A large high attenuation mass (arrows) seen in the left frontal lobe extends medially to the gray-white matter junction. Surrounding edema (black crescent-shaped area) is associated with the mass. Note the displacement of the left lateral ventricle to the right. Two images from his T1-weighted MR scan (Fig. 4–84, axial; Fig. 4–85, coronal) also show the large mass lesion in the left front lobe with mass effect. In addition, in Figure 4–86 (a lower-level axial slice), a second lesion (arrow) is seen in the right hemisphere without significant edema.

The finding of multiple brain masses often associated with edema should alert one to the possibility of brain metastases. Incidentally, malignant melanoma metastases are usually exceedingly bright on T1-weighted MR images, as in Figures 4–85 and 4–86. The presence of malignant melanoma brain metastases was confirmed by a brain biopsy. Mr. O'Leary began treatment with chemotherapy and radiation.

End of Case

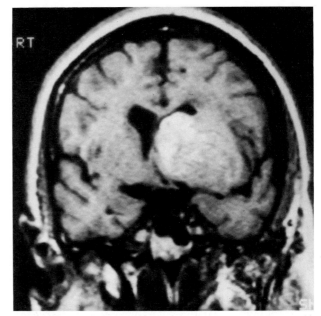

Figure 4–85   Mr. O'Leary, MRI scan, coronal image.

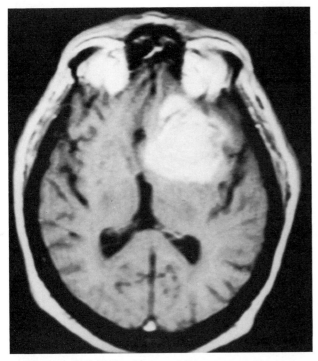

Figure 4–84   Philip O'Leary, MRI scan, axial image.

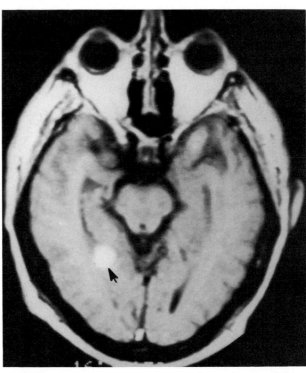

Figure 4–86   Mr. O'Leary, MRI scan, lower-level axial image.

Karen Weston: *(Continued from page 293)* CT demonstrates a densely enhancing, left, posterior temporal lobe mass. Notice the absence of surrounding edema, as compared with patients with brain metastases and a brain abscess. Also note that Ms. Weston's mass is broad based, against the inner table of the skull, giving one the impression that its epicenter might be the skull or meninges. What are your thoughts?

Continued Part D, page 339

Chad Gregory: *(Continued from page 293)* A left internal carotid arteriogram (Figs. 4–87 and 4–88) showed that the mass consists entirely of a tangled array of abnormal blood vessels, with massive arterial feeders from the middle cerebral artery (black arrowhead) and large veins (arrows) that drain the malformation into the superior sagittal sinus.

The therapeutic approaches to arteriovenous malformations are currently controversial and include surgical resection and percutaneous transcatheter embolization. Mr. Gregory is scheduled for embolotherapy next week.

End of Case

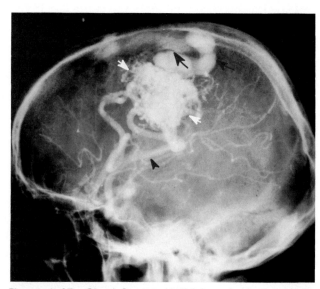

Figure 4–87 Chad Gregory, left internal carotid arteriogram.

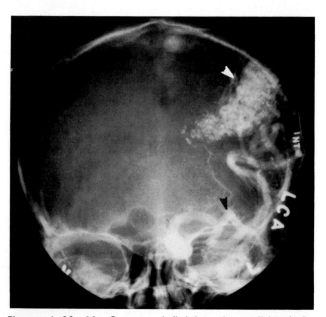

Figure 4–88 Mr. Gregory, left internal carotid arteriogram.

Paul Robertson: *(Continued from page 294)* His PA chest radiograph shows overaeration consistent with chronic obstructive pulmonary disease (see Fig. 4–46). The right side of the superior mediastinal contour is irregular and prominent, raising the possibility of a mediastinal mass. A contrast-enhanced CT scan would be the next step in the evaluation of this patient with mediastinal widening. However, because of the strong clinical suggestion of vascular involvement of the superior vena cava, a superior vena cavagram would have to follow the CT to demonstrate vascular occlusion. In addition to having been a smoker for many years, you find that your patient has also had long-standing diabetes with nephrosclerosis. Therefore, he would be at risk for contrast-enhanced CT. What other imaging methods can you think of that would define the mediastinum including the vascular structures without contrast?

Continued Part D, page 340.

Denise Morton: *(Continued from page 295)* Figure 4–48 is a PA view that shows a mass overlying the left hilar region. The left lung volume is diminished. The left hilum is displaced upwards, and the trachea is shifted slightly to the left. The mediastinum is also shifted slightly to the left, and the left diaphragm is minimally elevated. There is increased density in the left upper lung field, compared with the right, suggestive of a left upper lobe collapse or atelectasis. The lateral view confirms left upper lobe collapse. Figure 4–49 shows that the major fissure (arrows) is displaced anteriorly and the density anterior to it is the collapsed left upper lobe. The left lower lobe is hyperexpanded because of compensatory overaeration. What caused the left upper lobe collapse? How would you proceed?

Continued Part D, page 341.

Joe Bianti: *(Continued from page 294)* The esophagram shows an irregular narrowing of the distal esophagus. The pattern of irregularity did not change during the entire examination. The esophagus seemed fixed, nonmovable, and nondistensible. The findings suggest a carcinoma. A benign stricture is usually associated with smooth narrowing and shorter length. Inflammatory esophagitis is far less likely. On endoscopic biopsy, this patient had an infiltrating squamous cell carcinoma. A barium esophagram only shows the esophageal lumen. It is not possible to determine from the esophagram the involvement of the esophageal wall and tissues surrounding the esophagus. How would you image the esophageal wall and its surroundings?

Continued Part D, page 341.

Bruce Gunzel: *(Continued from page 296)* Figure 4–50 shows a normal left kidney with the normal left renal contour, calyces, and renal pelvis. On the right side, only one upper pole calyx is visualized. The rest are not seen, and there is a suggestion of a mass inferolaterally.

This appearance is suggestive of a tumor more than a cyst. A cyst would more likely displace calyces, rather than completely obliterate them. Therefore, from the intravenous urogram, renal neoplasm is the more likely diagnosis. What would you do next?

Continued Part D, page 343.

Ernest Jones: *(Continued from page 296)* The chest films are normal, without evidence of tuberculosis. No radiopaque renal calculi are seen on the plain abdominal film (see Fig. 4–17), although there are several incidental findings, including degenerative arthritis of the left hip, as well as vascular calcifications and phleboliths in the pelvis. To be certain that none of the phleboliths are distal ureteral calculi, compare the plain film with the contrast film (see Fig. 4–51). All the calcifications are external to the urinary tract.

The contrast film shows normal kidneys and ureters. In the bladder (Fig. 4–89), there is a large, round, lobulated filling defect that is nearly completely surrounded by a rim of contrast. The appearance is typical of a pedunculated bladder tumor, most likely carcinoma, which is attached to the right bladder floor by a thick pedicle. The bladder wall is thickened and flattened at the site of attachment, suggesting that the tumor is infiltrating the wall. The irregularities along the left dome of the bladder are also consistent with malignant infiltration. Frequently, bladder tumors will obstruct a ureteral orifice, producing hydroureter and hydronephrosis, although this did not occur here.

The appearance of bladder tumors may be mimicked by large blood clots and rarely by nonopaque stones within the bladder, as well as by a collection of gas in the rectum, which may be seen through a normal, contrast-filled bladder in the AP projection.

Benign tumors infrequently occur in the bladder. Secondary tumors arise by direct extension from the prostate gland, bowel, uterus, cervix, and ovary. How will you confirm your diagnosis of a primary bladder tumor?

Continued Part D, page 343.

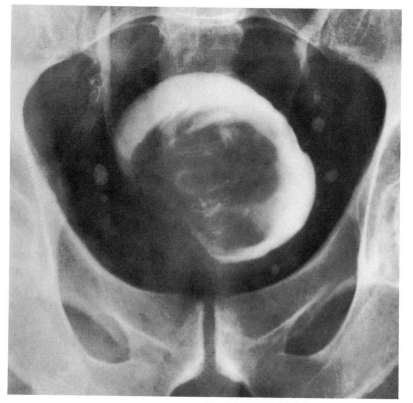

Figure 4–89 Mr. Jones, detail of bladder.

PATIENTS WITH PALLOR OR JAUNDICE (Continued from Part B, page 297)

Bertha Taylor: *(Continued from page 297)* The barium enema shows a bulky, irregular mass in the cecum (Fig. 4–90). Such a large, bulky mass and presenting symptoms of bleeding are highly suspicious for a neoplasm—an adenocarcinoma of the colon. How would you make a definite diagnosis and how would you determine the extent of Mrs. Taylor's disease, particularly in view of the fact that laboratory data showed abnormal liver function studies?

Continued Part D, page 344.

Juan Rivera: *(Continued from page 298)* Figure 4–55 shows dilated biliary ducts within the liver. These are branching hypodense structures (arrowheads). On Figure 4–92, at a lower level, the pancreatic mass in the area of the head of the pancreas (M), the cause of this patient's jaundice, is identified. Notice the moderately dilated gallbladder (G) secondary to biliary obstruction. This finding corresponds to a classic physical finding of a mass in a deeply jaundiced patient, the so-called Courvoisier's gallbladder. How would you diagnose Mr. Rivera's problem and how would you treat his condition?

Continued Part D, page 344.

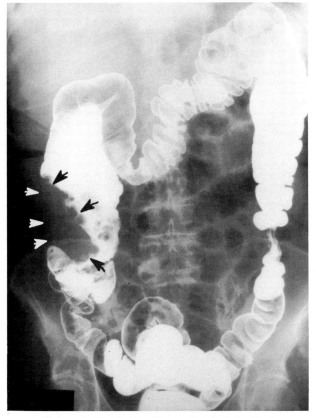

Figure 4–90   Bertha Taylor, barium enema.

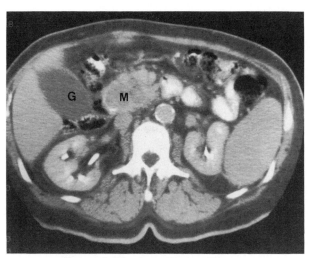

Figure 4–92   Juan Rivera, CT scan.

Adele Grabet: *(Continued from page 297)* You will want to search for possible metastatic disease, and because gastric cancers often spread locally to nearby lymph nodes, you would like to visualize the perigastric area as well. You will request a CT scan of the abdomen. What does Figure 4–91 show?

Continued Part D, page 344.

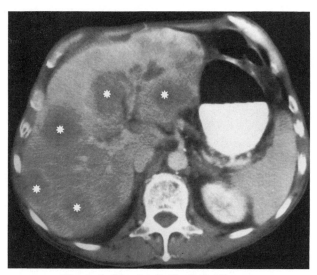

Figure 4–91   Adele Grabet, CT scan.

Barbara Crane: *(Continued from page 299)* Figure 4–56 is an AP view of Ms. Crane's knee that shows a large lytic lesion in the proximal portion of the lateral tibia extending to the end of the bone. This lesion is fairly well circumscribed, contains no calcifications, and seems to have expanded and thinned the bony cortex, making it prone to develop a pathologic fracture. A conventional tomogram (Figure 4–93) shows this lesion in better detail. In addition, it shows a depressed fracture of the tibial plateau (arrows). This fracture does account for Ms. Crane's acute sudden onset of pain. Could a CT scan of this area be useful?

Continued Part D, page 345.

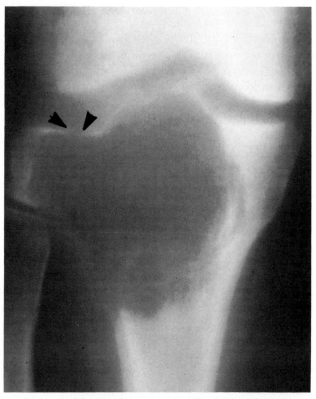

Figure 4–93 Ms. Crane, conventional tomograph.

WOMAN WITH A BREAST MASS (Continued from Part B, page 300)

Abby Xavier: *(Continued from page 300)* Breast cancer usually spreads to the lungs, liver, brain, and abdominal organs as well as to axillary lymph nodes. The plain chest radiograph, bone scan, and CT scans of the brain, chest, and abdomen were normal. Mrs. Xavier underwent a right mastectomy and did well. However, two years later, a CT scan of the abdomen was performed (Fig. 4–94), and irregular lesions within the liver were suggestive of metastases. Note also the breast prosthesis on the right side. Figure 4–95 is a lower cut through the midliver area that shows additional multiple liver lesions, which on biopsy with ultrasound guidance, showed metastatic breast cancer consistent with the primary breast lesion. Following chemotherapy, the CT scan of the abdomen became normal for at least two years.

End of Case

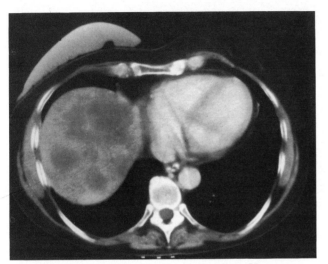

Figure 4–94 Abby Xavier, abdominal CT scan.

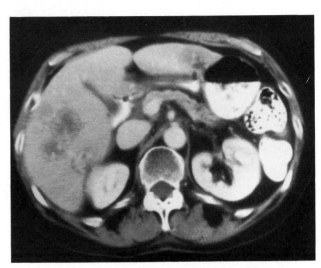

Figure 4–95 Mrs. Xavier, midhepatic CT scan.

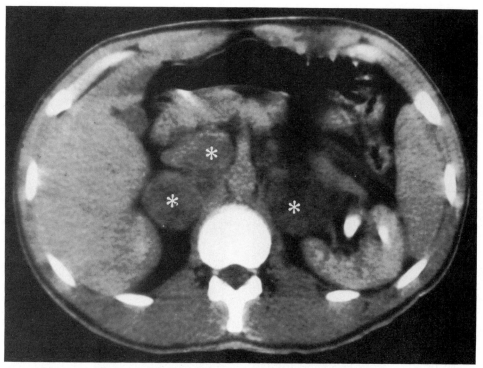

Figure 4–96   Jose Garcia, lower abdominal CT scan.

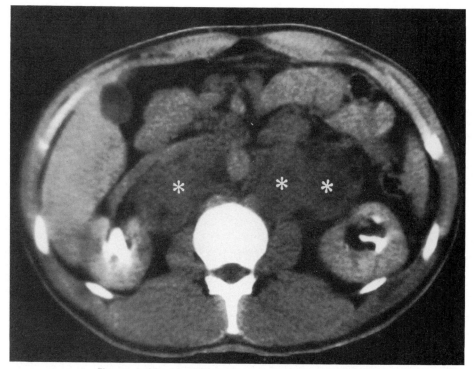

Figure 4–97   Mr. Garcia, lower abdominal CT scan.

Jose Garcia: Testicular neoplasms usually metastasize via the testicular lymphatics, which follow the courses of the testicular veins. These veins drain into the para-aortic lymph nodes at the level of the renal veins. Therefore, an abdominal CT scan is what you should request in order to search for para-aortic lymphadenopathy. Figure 4–96 shows large, inhomogeneous, predominantly hypodense masses in the retroperitoneum (asterisks). These masses represent retroperitoneal adenopathy. Figure 4–97 shows larger abnormal lymph nodes at a slightly lower level. Notice the displacement of both kidneys laterally and the displacement of the right renal vein superiorly, as well as the lifting of the aorta off the vertebral body. Figure 4–98 shows an abdominal film that was taken following CT and shows marked displacement of the kidneys and ureters laterally. CT scans of the chest and bone also should be done to search for possible metastases.

This patient had orchiectomy and pelvic and retroperitoneal lymph node dissection. A seminoma was the tissue diagnosis at these sites. The patient was placed on chemotherapy and is doing well three years following initial diagnosis.

End of Case

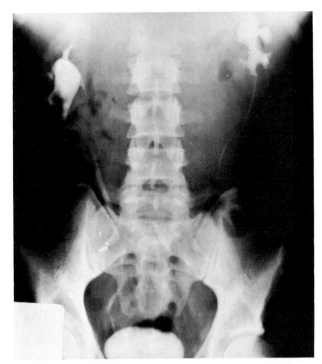

Figure 4–98 Mr. Garcia, abdominal radiograph.

Part D

PATIENTS WITH COUGH (Continued from Part C, page 304)

Febrile Drug Addict with Fever and Heart Murmur (Companion Case to Brian Seldinger)

Bilateral peripheral ill-defined nodular opacities are present. On the CT scan shown in Figure 4–99, some of these nodules are demonstrated in more detail with a vessel (arrows) entering such a nodule. The roentgen findings are highly suggestive of septic pulmonary infarcts.

In drug addicts, intravenously injected material travels to the right atrium and via the tricuspid valve into the right ventricle and out into the pulmonary arteries and peripheral lung fields. Most of the time bacterial endocarditis is also present.

End of Case

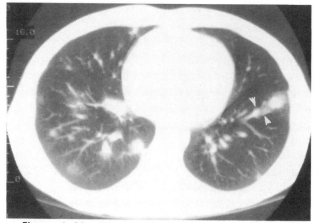

Figure 4–99   CT scan of the patient in Figure 4–64.

JOHN DOE (Continued from Part C, page 303)

Figure 4–100 at the renal level shows a normal right psoas muscle (P), and arrows point to air pockets in the left psoas muscle. Figure 4–101 at an infrarenal level demonstrates this psoas abscess with a larger, confluent cavity. These CT findings suggest a psoas abscess associated with spinal tuberculosis. He had more intense antituberculous chemotherapy with significant improvement.

End of Case

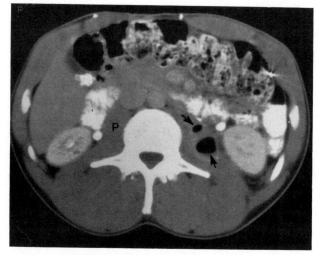

Figure 4–100   John Doe, CT scan.

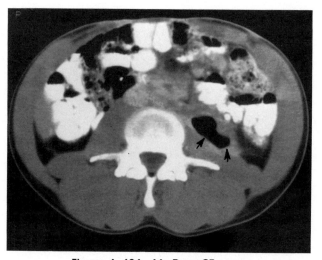

Figure 4–101   Mr. Doe, CT scan.

PATIENT WITH SHORTNESS OF BREATH (SOB) (Continued from Part C, page 305)

Paul O'Grady: *(Continued from page 305)* Multiple pulmonary nodules may arise from liver, kidney, testes, head, neck, and primary skin cancers. Do you want to do an upper GI series, a barium enema, an IVU, an abdominal CT scan (the traditional primary site hunt) and possibly not even come close to the diagnosis? You want to get to the actual pathologic process, and a percutaneous lung biopsy is what you should be thinking about as the definitive method of diagnosis. However, *you* notice the subcutaneous nodule in the right chest. This is the simplest and the most approachable lesion. There-

fore, this one was biopsied and the pathologic study showed metastatic melanoma. Upon further questioning, Mr. O'Grady mentioned that one summer between his senior year in high school and freshman year in college, he was a lifeguard on the beach and used no sun protection. You find an ulcerated mole on his back, which is biopsied and proved to be a melanoma. He received chemotherapy with some temporary improvement.

End of Case

PATIENT WITH ACUTE BACK PAIN (Continued from Part C, page 305)

Matilda Mason: *(Continued from page 305)* The change in the contour of the superior mediastinum with widening should make you suspect the possibility of a mediastinal hematoma associated with a thoracic aortic aneurysm. Atherosclerotic and hypertensive aneurysms are the most common. Traumatic aneurysm may occur at the root of the aorta or just beyond the origin of the left subclavian artery. There is no history for any of the above. A mycotic aneurysm might be another possibility in view of the recent surgery as well as the elevated temperature in this patient. Therefore, you request a CT scan of the chest (Fig. 4–102). What do you think?

Continued Part E, page 346.

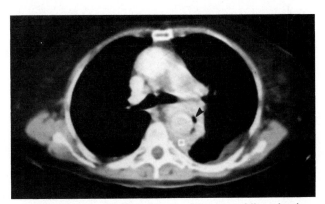

Figure 4–102 Matilda Mason, CT scan of the chest.

Lisa Morgan: *(Continued from page 306)* The barium enema is done because it is believed that a gentle but careful study of Ms. Morgan's colon, *in the absence of signs of perforation and peritonitis,* might be the most direct method of obtaining the diagnosis of inflammatory bowel disease. This would be particularly true if the barium enema showed ulcerations or an inflammatory mass. It was also believed that, should the barium enema be unrewarding, it would then be necessary to proceed with an upper GI series and small bowel study. In such a case it would be wise to do the barium enema first to rule out such other colonic diseases as ulcerative colitis, tuberculosis, and amebiasis, all of which may affect the cecum.

The barium enema is negative and the GI series and small bowel study are done two days later. The first film (Fig. 4–103), taken at 30 minutes, shows barium progressing through normal jejunum into midileum. The right lower quadrant is still suspiciously empty. The next film, at 60 minutes (Fig. 4–104), shows barium in terminal small bowel and just beginning to fill the cecum. What is abnormal?

Continued Part E, page 346.

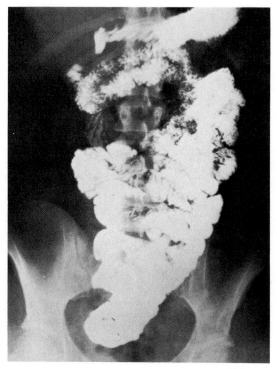

Figure 4–103 Lisa Morgan, 30-minute film.

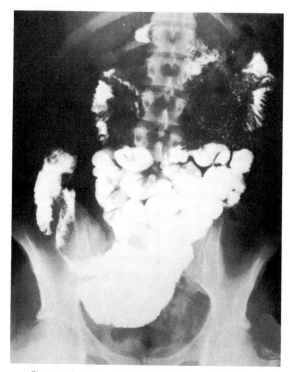

Figure 4–104 Ms. Morgan, 60-minute film.

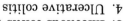

Figure 4–105 Pierre Claude, barium enema.

Pierre Claude: *(Continued from page 306)* After consultation with the radiologist and without any bowel preparation, you request an emergency barium enema to confirm what you by now strongly suspect to be the diagnosis. Here are the barium enema films (Figs. 4–105 and 4–106). Were you correct?

Continued Part E, page 347.

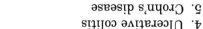

Figure 4–106 M. Claude, barium enema.

Name Five Causes of Diarrhea

Answer

1. Gastroenteritis
2. Ischemic colitis
3. Infectious colitis (salmonella, shigella, ameba)
4. Ulcerative colitis
5. Crohn's disease

Agnes Delarenzo: *(Continued from page 306)* Figures 4–107 and 4–108 are the CT sections of the upper abdomen on which you will notice within the liver a grapefruit-sized hypodense area (arrows) with multiple air pockets. This area represents a liver abscess. Why did Mrs. Delarenzo develop a liver abscess?

Continued Part E, page 348.

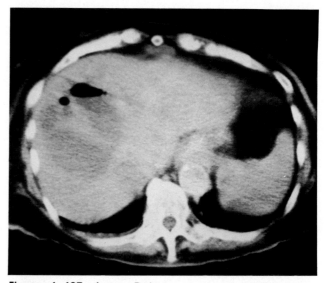

Figure 4–107 Agnes Delarenzo, upper abdominal CT scan.

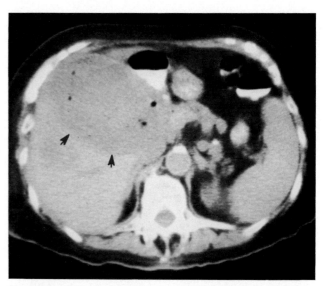

Figure 4–108 Mrs. Delarenzo, upper abdominal CT scan.

Leo Cleveland: *(Continued from page 306)* Figure 4–109 is a gallbladder ultrasound study that shows numerous tiny echogenic foci representing gallstones. Figure 4–110 is an ultrasound study of a very dilated common bile duct (asterisks) with a demonstrable stone in it (arrowhead).

With conservative supportive treatment of nasogastric suction and antibiotics, the patient improved significantly, with abatement of the abdominal and chest pain and marked decrease in the amylase level. Several weeks later, Mr. Cleveland underwent elective cholecystectomy, and calculi were found in both gallbladder and common bile duct.

End of Case

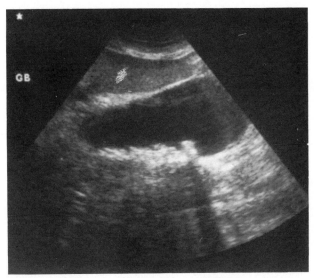

Figure 4–109 Leo Cleveland, gallbladder ultrasound study.

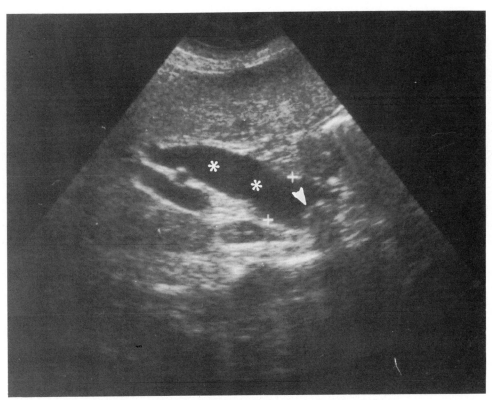

Figure 4–110 Mr. Cleveland, bile duct ultrasound study.

Harvey Conrad: *(Continued from page 306)* You request a gallbladder ultrasound.

Figure 4–111 is a transverse sonogram of Mr. Conrad's gallbladder. The gallbladder is recognized with ultrasound by its echo-free lumen and sac-like shape, but Mr. Conrad has several very echogenic stones at the bottom of his gallbladder (curved arrow) which produce an acoustic shadow below (straight arrows). Figure 4–112 is an ultrasound of a normal gallbladder.

Identifying gallstones on ultrasound is important; however, the symptoms may not be due to the gallstones. Sometimes, a nuclear medicine hepatobiliary scan can identify cholecystitis—inflammatory changes in gallbladder that may cause the symptoms. These two examinations—gallbladder ultrasound and hepatobiliary scan—can diagnose cholelithiasis and cholecystitis.

At cholecystectomy, several large stones were found in Mr. Conrad's gallbladder and he made a good recovery.

End of Case

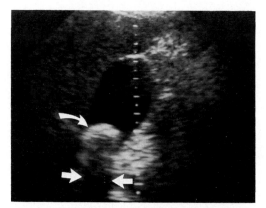

Figure 4–111 Harvey Conrad, sonogram.

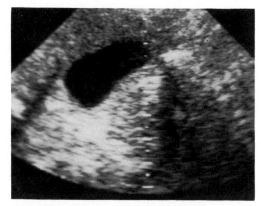

Figure 4–112 Normal sonogram of another patient.

Abner Lane: *(Continued from page 308)* The early and late films of the superior mesenteric arteriogram demonstrate extravasation of contrast medium in a sac-like structure in the right colon (Figs. 4–113 and 4–114). It appears that Mr. Lane has actively bleeding diverticulosis. However, other bleeding pathologic lesions in the colon may produce a similar angiographic pattern. (In addition, he has a "replaced hepatic artery," a congenital variation, arising from the superior mesenteric artery, black arrow.)

Now that you have *located* the bleeding site, how will you stop the bleeding?

Continued Part E, page 349.

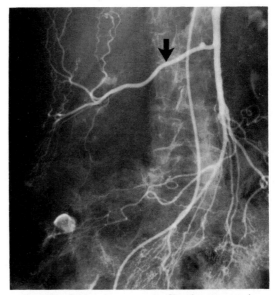

Figure 4–113 Abner Lane, early film from superior mesenteric arteriogram.

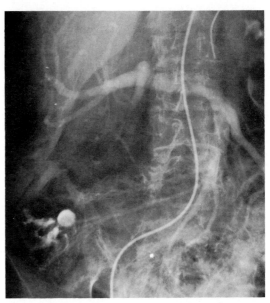

Figure 4–114 Mr. Lane, late venous phase from superior mesenteric ateriogram.

Ivan Picot: *(Continued from page 308)* A ventilation and perfusion lung scan is the next recommended examination. The ventilation scan is done first. This consists of inhalation of radioactive gas (xenon 133) followed by posterior images of the lungs, which are taken with a gamma camera. Figure 4–115 shows the posterior ventilation scan, which is normal. Next Mr. Picot had a perfusion scan; Figure 4–116 is also a posterior view. This scan involved injection of radioactive particles (macroaggregated albumin particles tagged with radioactive technetium 99). These are embolized intravenously into .1% of the millions of pulmonary arterioles. Images of the lungs are obtained with the gamma camera in various projections over every portion of the lung. Figure 4–116, a posterior view, shows virtually complete absence of perfusion to the right lung with a normal perfusion of the left lung. Certainly, the findings of the chest radiograph, the normal ventilation scan, and the clearly abnormal perfusion scan confirm the diagnosis of pulmonary embolism. Heparinization would be the appropriate treatment. However, in this patient there may be an alternative method of treatment. Why? What is the method of treatment?

Continued Part E, page 350.

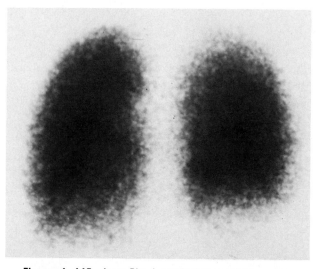

Figure 4–115 Ivan Picot, posterior ventilation scan.

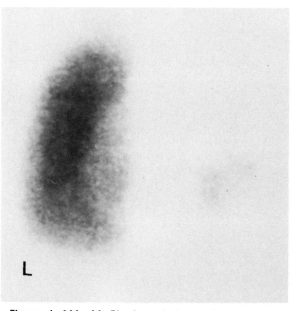

Figure 4–116 Mr. Picot, posterior perfusion scan.

PATIENT FROM THE ROAD (Continued from Part C, page 311)

Darryl Halston: *(Continued from page 311)* Simple linear liver lacerations without hemoperitoneum generally heal on conservative management. You would, of course, admit the patient to the hospital and carefully monitor the hematocrit and vital signs for evidence of further bleeding. In addition, you would request a follow-up CT scan several days later and prior to discharge.

Mr. Halston did remain stable, and the liver scan done on his fourth hospital day showed no evidence of further bleeding. Figure 4–117 is a repeat CT scan one month later, taken at the same level, but now showing complete healing of the liver laceration. Because Mr. Halston was more cooperative, the quality of the last CT scan is much improved. This scan was performed with both intravenous and oral contrast media. Note the large collection of contrast material in the stomach—that is normal.

CT has proved helpful in identifying trauma patients whose injuries are so minor that surgery may not be necessary for their management. Unnecessary surgery is then avoided. It is also reassuring to be able to perform follow-up CT to confirm that healing is taking place.

Incidentally, CT scans assist in diagnosing a variety of parenchymal organ injuries in the trauma patient. Figure 4–118 is a four-year-old child with a subcapsular hematoma of the liver suffered during a fall down a flight of stairs. Figure 4–119 is the CT scan of a ten-year-old child who skated into a stone wall and suffered a pancreatic fracture (arrows). Figure 4–120 is the CT scan of a 14-year-old patient with a shattered kidney suffered during a bicycle accident. Note the extravasation of opacified urine anteriorly (asterisk) and the kidney parenchymal laceration (arrowhead) and perirenal hematoma (solid circles).

End of Case

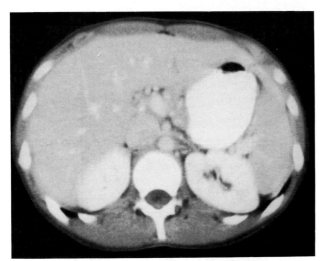

Figure 4–117 Darryl Halston, repeat CT scan.

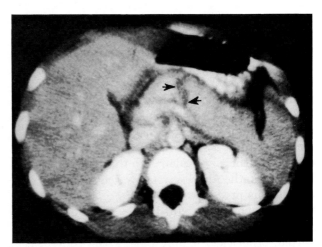

Figure 4–119 CT scan of child with a pancreatic fracture.

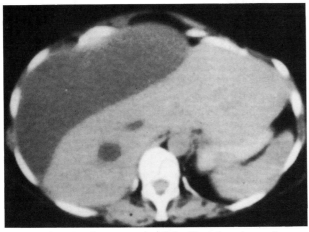

Figure 4–118 CT scan of child with a liver hematoma.

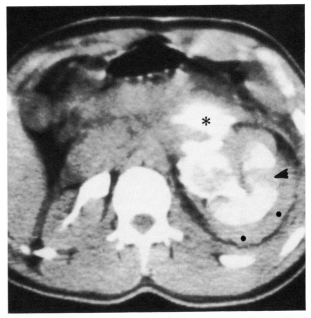

Figure 4–120 CT scan of a 14-year-old patient with a shattered kidney.

Priscilla Lazardi: *(Continued from page 315)* Pheochromocytomas occur most commonly in the adrenal medulla; however, they may also occur anywhere along the sympathic ganglionic chain, either in the chest or in the abdomen, and frequently they are multiple. Occasionally, they may even arise in the urinary bladder or in the pelvis in the so-called organ of Zuckerkandl. CT scans of the abdomen and chest including the pelvis are the most common methods of examination to demonstrate pheochromocytomas, particularly in the adrenal glands. Figure 4–125 is a CT scan of the abdomen without intravenous contrast at the level of the adrenals. What do you think?

Continued Part E, page 351.

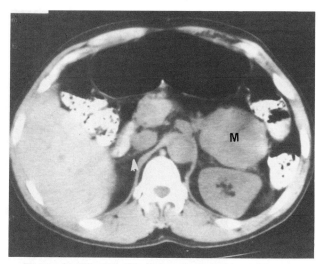

Figure 4–125 Priscilla Lazardi, abdominal CT scan.

Mary Pastone: *(Continued from page 315)* Initial blood studies show her to have a severe normocytic anemia. The smear shows pronounced rouleaux formation and the sedimentation rate is increased. The laboratory also reports hyperproteinemia, serum calcium 14.8, and normal phosphorus and alkaline phosphatase.

The next day the serum electrophoretic pattern is returned, which was asked for by the attending, showing the presence of hyperglobulinemia with striking elevation of both the gamma and beta fractions. There is Bence Jones protein in the urine and the skeletal survey and bone scan are compatible with multiple myeloma. Is the lateral skull film in keeping with this diagnosis? (Fig. 4–126.)

Yes. It is important to remember that although 90 per cent of all patients with multiple myeloma have bone pain at some time, 5 per cent never show

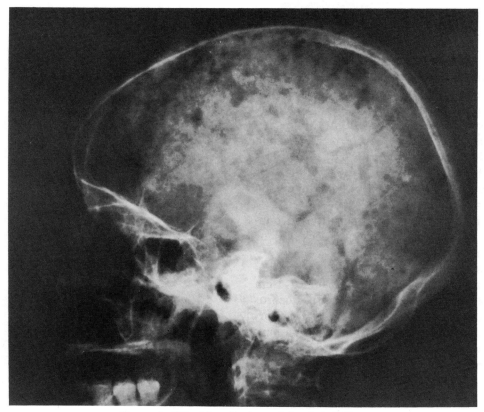

Figure 4–126 Mary Pastone, lateral skull film.

any radiographic changes at all, and a great many smolder along with films that are indistinguishable from osteoporosis for some time before the spotty, punched-out, smooth-margined lesions that are so characteristic develop. Remember that 40 to 50 per cent of the bone must be lost before the radiologic appearance itself is very impressive. Of course, the diagnosis of simple osteoporosis is excluded by finding the pathognomonic proteins of myeloma in serum and urine, *if* one thinks of looking for them.

For this reason, too, patients with a tentative diagnosis of osteoporosis in this age group probably deserve bone density determinations rather than just spine films. It is often easier to be sure of punched-out lesions in bones (like the skull and ribs) where the cortex is smooth and flat than in complex bones like the vertebrae. Mrs. Pastone's humeral fracture was, of course, pathologic.

End of Case

PATIENTS WITH NEUROLOGICAL DEFICITS (Continued from Part C, page 318)

Karen Weston: *(Continued from page 318)* A small, slow-growing benign meningioma is highly suggested by the insidious onset of symptoms, absence of findings on physical examination, location on CT scan, and absence of surrounding edema. A magnetic resonance (MRI) scan was performed, and this examination also confirms the presence of a broad-based mass with essentially no surrounding edema. The mass is low in signal strength on the T2-weighted axial image (Fig. 4–127, axial plane), but after IV gadolinium (Fig. 4–128, coronal plane), the lesion brightly enhances and is homogeneous in distribution of enhancement. You can see that the mass is separate from the skull, which appeared black at MRI because of absent signal. The location, apparently arising from the meninges, and strong enhancement with gadolinium, are typical of meningioma.

Arteriography is often performed on patients with meningioma. Which arteries would you expect to supply this lesion?

Continued Part E, page 352.

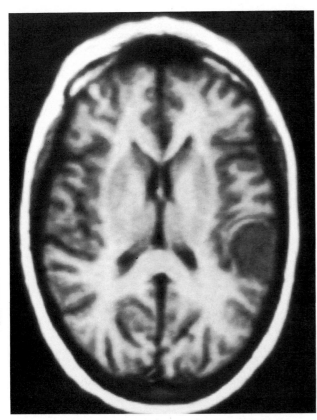

Figure 4–127 Karen Weston, MRI scan, axial plane.

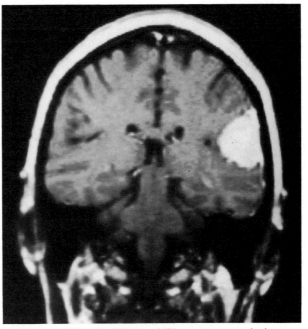

Figure 4–128 Ms. Weston, MRI scan, coronal plane.

Paul Robertson: *(Continued from page 319)* MRI examination shows vascular structures because freely flowing blood gives rise to no signal and vessels therefore appear black, whereas a tumor mass has certain signal characteristics and is grayish. Figures 4–129 to 4–130 show coronal sections from anterior to posterior. Anteriorly, the ascending aorta and the arch of the aorta (asterisk) are seen. Just to the right of the aortic arch, a grayish mass (M) is present. This mass can be seen to better advantage on Figure 4–147 showing the superior extent of the mass, which is compressing and invading the superior vena cava (asterisk). Incidentally, notice the liver lesion. Establishing a diagnosis of a mediastinal mass may often be accomplished with transthoracic percutaneous mediastinal biopsy. In this case that procedure would be contraindicated. Can you think of a reason why, and how would you make a diagnosis on this patient?

Continued Part E, page 352.

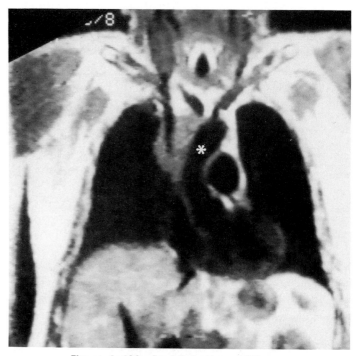

Figure 4–129 Paul Robertson, MRI scan.

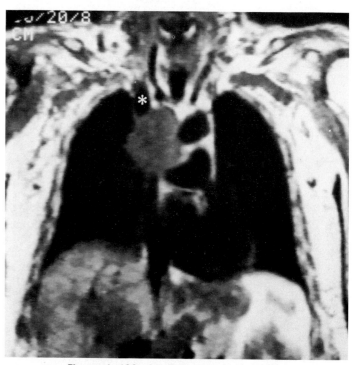

Figure 4–130 Mr. Robertson, MRI scan.

Joe Bianti: *(Continued from page 319)* You want a CT scan. Figure 4–131 is through the level of the dome of the liver and spleen and shows a large, bulky mass extending to the gastroesophageal junction (arrows). The size of the mass was not apparent from the esophagram, nor was its widely infiltrating nature. Note also at least two enlarged retrocrural lymph nodes (black dots). This patient did not have hepatic metastases, nor did he have any evidence of metastases aside from the retrocrural ones. Mr. Bianti received radiation therapy with improvement of symptoms and subsequently had surgery. He had two more winning seasons with one of his boxers.

End of Case

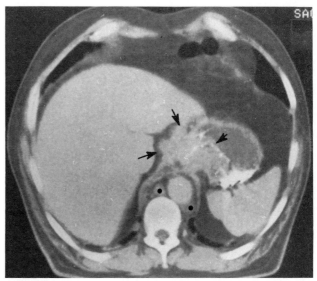

Figure 4–131 Joe Bianti, CT scan through the liver and spleen.

Denise Morton: *(Continued from page 319)* A CT scan at the level of the aortic arch shows a triangular soft tissue density—the collapsed left upper lobe plastered against the anterior chest wall and mediastinum (arrows, Fig. 4–132). At the level of the main pulmonary artery (Fig. 4–133), the left upper lobe bronchus is obstructed by a small intrabronchial mass (arrow). The mediastinum and chest wall are normal. The CT appearance is highly suggestive of an intrabronchial lesion of the left upper lobe bronchus, probably a squamous cell carcinoma that has caused atelectasis of the left upper lobe. Mrs. Morton had bronchoscopy and a lesion was noted in the left upper lobe bronchus causing the obstruction. This lesion was biopsied and was found to be a squamous cell carcinoma. Cigarette smoking is the leading cause of primary lung cancer.

The CT scan of the pelvis also shows a soft tissue mass in the subcutaneous fat just behind the gluteus maximus muscle (arrow, Fig. 4–134). On percutaneous biopsy, the lesion was found to be a metastatic squamous cell carcinoma. On a contrast-enhanced CT scan of the brain (Fig. 4–135), a ring-enhancing mass is present in the right posterior-parietal area with surrounding hypodense edema (arrows). This lesion is highly suggestive of a metastatic lesion. An abdominal CT scan showed liver and left adrenal metastases (asterisks), later confirmed by CT-guided biopsies (Fig. 4–136) to be squamous cell carcinoma. Because of the presence of extensive distant metastases, Mrs. Morton was treated with chemotherapy, improved, and returned to her CPA firm for at least two more seasons.

End of Case

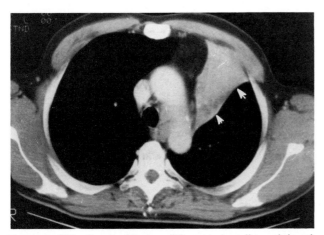

Figure 4–132 Denise Morton, CT scan at aortic arch level.

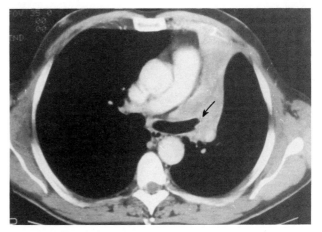

Figure 4–133 Mrs. Morton, CT scan at the level of the main pulmonary artery level.

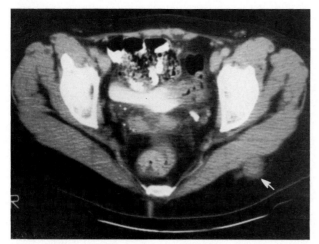

Figure 4–134   Mrs. Morton, pelvic CT scan.

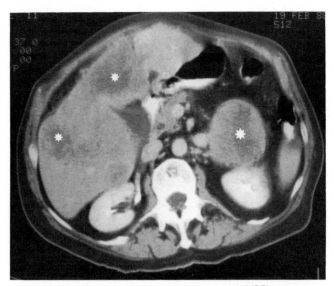

Figure 4–136   Mrs. Morton, abdominal CT scan.

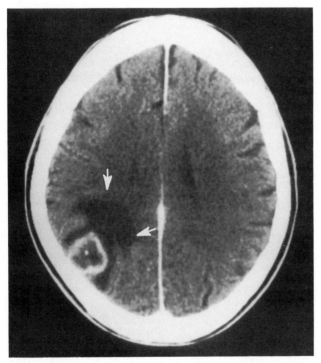

Figure 4–135   Mrs. Morton, brain CT scan.

Bruce Gunzel: *(Continued from page 320)* Ultrasound examination is helpful to distinguish a cyst from a solid tumor. However, on the evidence of the intravenous urogram, a tumor was more likely. Therefore, CT is the more appropriate examination in this case. CT scans at the renal levels show a normal left kidney (Figs. 4–137 and 4–138). A large, bulky, irregular mass is occupying the right kidney. In Figure 4–137, soft tissue density in the enlarged right renal vein (black arrows) is suggestive of invasion by tumor. Notice the normal-sized left renal vein (white arrows). In Figure 4–138, a hypodense area within the inferior vena cava is suggestive of caval invasion by tumor (asterisk).

In order to confirm your impression of vena caval invasion, a more definitive procedure must be done. What do you think the procedure or procedures would be?

Continued Part E, page 353.

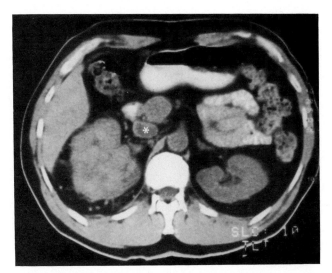

Figure 4–138 Mr. Gunzel, renal CT scan.

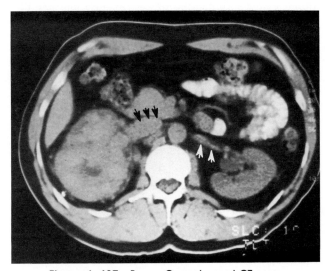

Figure 4–137 Bruce Gunzel, renal CT scan.

Ernest Jones: *(Continued from page 320)* You refer the patient for cystoscopy. A large tumor almost completely filling the bladder is identified. Biopsy is interpreted as transitional cell carcinoma.

Bone scan and liver CT are negative for metastatic disease. A pelvic CT scan confirms invasion of the bladder wall. A radical cystectomy with pelvic lymph node dissection is performed, and a bladder is constructed from the cecum. Postoperatively, the patient does well and is discharged on the nineteenth day.

By the way, any patient with hematuria should have cystoscopy, regardless of whether the intravenous urogram (IVU) is normal. Remember that the IVU has limited value in examining the bladder.

End of Case

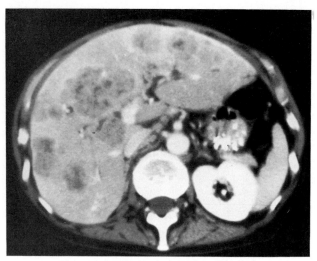

Figure 4–139 Bertha Taylor, CT scan.

Bertha Taylor: *(Continued from page 321)* Mrs. Taylor had a colonoscopy, and a bulky lesion seen in the cecum was biopsied and found to be an adenocarcinoma. Figure 4–139 is a CT scan of the abdomen through the liver that shows innumerable mass lesions that are inhomogeneous, mostly with central hypodense areas and perhaps some enhancement. Percutaneous aspiration biopsy showed metastatic colonic carcinoma. Mrs. Taylor had resection of the right side of the colon and received chemotherapy. Several months later she returned to her job and once again took care of your lunch.

End of Case

Adele Grabet: *(Continued from page 321)* CT image through the liver shows innumerable irregular inhomogeneous abnormal masses in the liver (see Fig. 4–91), consistent with extensive metastatic disease (asterisks). Notice that the gastric lesion is not seen on this section. Because proof of the presence of metastatic disease in the liver is essential for treatment planning, Mrs. Grabet had a percutaneous liver aspiration by the radiologist that showed a cellular pattern similar to that on the endoscopic biopsy from the stomach. With the combination of surgery and chemotherapy, the patient significantly improved for a period of about eight months, after which she succumbed to extensive distant metastases.

End of Case

Juan Rivera: *(Continued from page 321)* Most likely the mass in the area of the head of the pancreas is a carcinoma, although occasionally focal pancreatitis may have a similar appearance. Mr. Rivera had a CT-guided percutaneous biopsy of the mass (an interventional procedure) that showed an adenocarcinoma of the pancreas. He underwent percutaneous biliary drainage and eventual stent placement for the relief of the jaundice. With the stent, the drainage of the bile was accomplished directly into the duodenum. He went back to the night club for several more months. However, 18 months later he died of extensive liver metastases.

End of Case

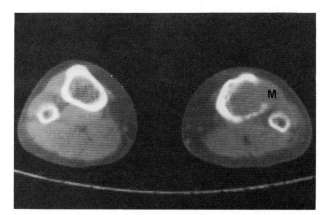

Figure 4–140

Barbara Crane: *(Continued from page 322)* Yes, CT would be very helpful in staging the extent of the tumor and would aid in the differential diagnostic considerations. Figure 4–140 shows a CT scan of both tibias. In addition to the destructive lesion on the affected side, an associated soft tissue component can be identified (M). A bone cyst would contain fluid rather than soft tissue density material and would not be associated with an accompanying soft tissue mass. CT does define exquisitely not only the bony details but also soft tissue abnormalities that could not be appreciated on the plain film. What kind of bony lesion is this?

Continued Part E, page 353.

Part E

PATIENT WITH ACUTE BACK PAIN (Continued from Part D, page 327)

Matilda Mason: *(Continued from page 327)* The CT scan of the chest shows, at the level of the carina, the descending portion of the aorta with air in the wall and an associated soft tissue mass around the aorta (see Fig. 4–102). The small left pleural effusion is also evident. The combination of the patient's history, the mediastinal widening, and the air in the aortic wall is highly suggestive of a mycotic aneurysm. Her blood cultures are reported positive for an *Enterobacter* organism, and she was started on IV antibiotics. How would you confirm the exact location and nature of this aneurysm?

Continued Part F, page 354.

PATIENTS WITH DIARRHEA (Continued from Part D, page 328)

Lisa Morgan: *(Continued from page 328)* The terminal ileum is abnormal (Fig. 4–141, a detail film). The last six inches show irregular narrowing and an abnormal "cobblestone" appearance of the mucosa due to criss-crossing ulcers and fissures that define islands of hyperplastic mucosa. There is also slight proximal dilatation of the ileum, and there is an increase in soft tissue density on either side of the terminal ileum due to surrounding inflammatory mass. It displaces adjacent small bowel loops to the left. The slightly dilated distal small bowel and the inflammatory "mass" could both be at least suspected on the initial plain film.

These x-ray findings are characteristic of terminal ileitis (regional ileitis or granulomatous ileitis), a disease that affects young adults, and presents as a febrile illness with cramps and either diarrhea or constipation. Gross bleeding is rare and there is a significant incidence of concomitant or future involvement of the colon by the same process. In fact, this patient, who initially does well on antibiotics and a low-roughage diet, returns nine months later with involvement of the cecum and ascending colon.

End of Case

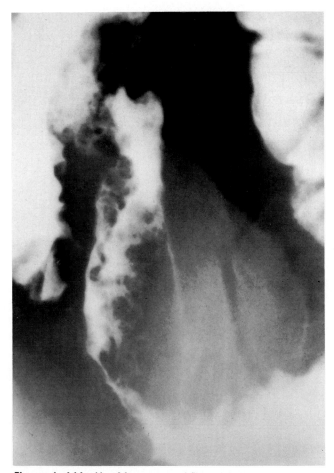

Figure 4–141 Lisa Morgan, spot film of the terminal ileum.

Pierre Claude: *(Continued from page 329)* The pre- and postevacuation films from the barium enema show that barium has outlined normal colon up to a point just proximal to the hepatic flexure. No further passage of barium into the right colon or cecum has occurred. The large gas- and feces-filled structure is still seen occupying most of the left side of the abdomen.

This picture is just about classic for a full-blown cecal volvulus. A cecal volvulus may occur, usually presenting as an acute large-bowel obstruction, in patients who have a very mobile cecum. This mobility is due to incomplete rotation of the colon, or to failure of fixation of the ascending colon after proper rotation. These rotation events are normally completed successfully in the twelfth fetal week.

Volvulus most often occurs in males in middle or late life. If the mobile cecum should become twisted on itself, as it did in Monsieur Claude's case, it then gradually distends, with gas passing into it from normal small bowel. The distension becomes so great that the cecum moves out of its usual position in the right lower abdomen and is forced into the mid- or left abdomen. The plain film of the abdomen will show the hugely dilated air shadow of the cecum in an unexpected position. There is almost always a fair amount of gas in the small bowel, whereas the colon distal to the twist is empty. A barium enema will confirm the suspected diagnosis by revealing a normal distal colon up to the point of twist. The column of barium frequently ends abruptly with a funnel-shaped configuration that represents the actual point of twist. The air-distended cecum, and often a portion of the ascending colon, will be seen to occupy an abnormal position in the mid- or left abdomen (Fig. 4–142). You schedule the patient for surgery. A right colectomy is performed.

End of Case

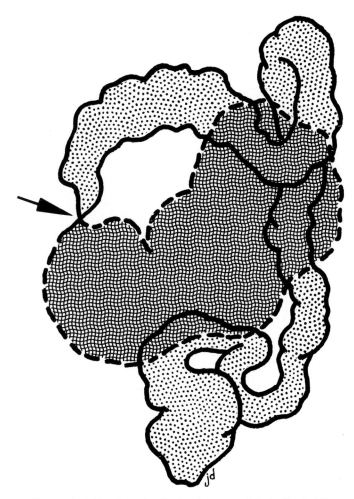

Figure 4–142 Cecal volvulus (arrow points to the twist).

Agnes Delarenzo: *(Continued from page 330)* A liver abscess may develop in a patient who has recently undergone abdominal surgery. A perforated appendicitis or diverticulitis may lead to the development of a liver abscess, but Mrs. Delarenzo had no history to suggest any of these. She has not reported any travel history around the Mediterranean to you, where amebic abscess or echinococcal cyst may occur that may look like what you saw on the CT scan. Perforated gastric or duodenal ulcers may lead to the development of a liver abscess, but she has no such history of ulcers. Metastatic lesions in the liver may grow to a large size and break down into an abscess. She does not give any history to you of a known primary cancer. Finally, acute cholecystitis with gangrene and perforation may result in a liver abscess.

Upon extensive questioning, you find that Mrs. Delarenzo has had gallstones for many years and has had, off and on, some right upper abdominal discomfort, particularly in the last few weeks. You confirm Mrs. Delarenzo's problem with gallbladder ultrasound, which shows gallstones, a thickened gallbladder wall, and pericholecystic fluid. Subsequently, a hepatobiliary scan demonstrates no radioactive material within the gallbladder and is consistent with an acute cystic duct obstruction. The etiology of the liver abscess therefore is perforation of an acutely inflamed gallbladder into the liver parenchyma.

Treatment consisted of an interventional procedure, a percutaneous abscess drainage with CT guidance, and antibiotics. Several weeks later she had elective cholecystectomy.

End of Case

Abner Lane: *(Continued from page 333)* Hemorrhage can be stopped in more than 85 per cent of colonic lesions actively bleeding from arterial sites with intraarterial infusion of vasopressin (at 0.2 to 0.4 U/min for 24 to 48 hours). The radiologist secures the angiographic catheter in place, with its tip in the superior mesenteric artery, and begins an infusion of vasopressin. Twenty minutes later a repeat arteriogram shows good vasoconstrictor effect and no further bleeding (Fig. 4–143). Clinically the patient stopped bleeding and the catheter was removed after 48 hours of vasopressin therapy. Do you send the patient home, or does he require further study?

Continued Part F, page 354.

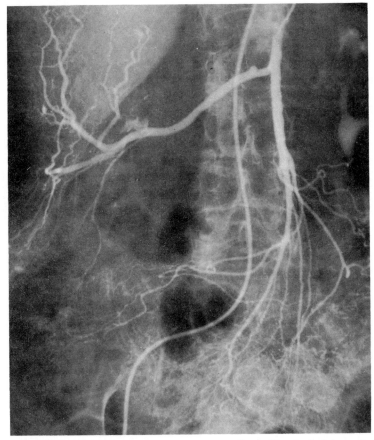

Figure 4–143   Abner Lane, repeat superior mesenteric arteriogram after a 20-minute intra-arterial infusion of vasopressin.

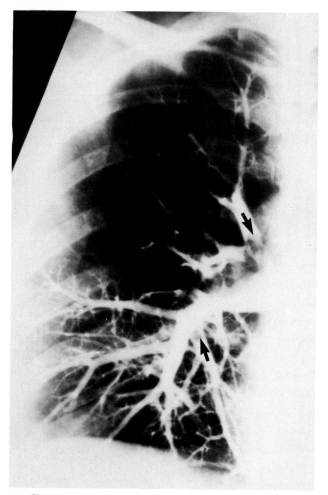

Ivan Picot: *(Continued from page 334)* Because of Mr. Picot's recent brain surgery, heparinization is contraindicated. Therefore, he underwent a confirmatory pulmonary arteriogram followed by an insertion of an inferior vena cava filter. Figure 4–144, the pulmonary arteriogram, shows filling defects of the pulmonary arteries and markedly decreased perfusion in the RUL.

He recovered uneventfully from brain surgery and pulmonary emboli.

End of Case

Figure 4–144   Ivan Picot, pulmonary arteriogram.

Priscilla Lazardi: (*Continued from page 338*) An approximately 5 × 5 cm mass in the suprarenal region on the left side is apparent (see Fig. 4–125, M). This finding is consistent with a pheochromocytoma. The arrow is pointing to a normal portion of the right adrenal gland. At the midrenal level, in Figure 4–145, are two smaller round masses (asterisks), which also proved to be pheochromocytomas at surgery. This patient had a retroperitoneal exploration with a left-sided adrenalectomy and removal of the masses that were described at CT. There was a careful communication between radiologist and surgeon *during* the surgical procedure, and only following removal of all the masses did the patient's blood pressure return to normal. She was permanently cured.

End of Case

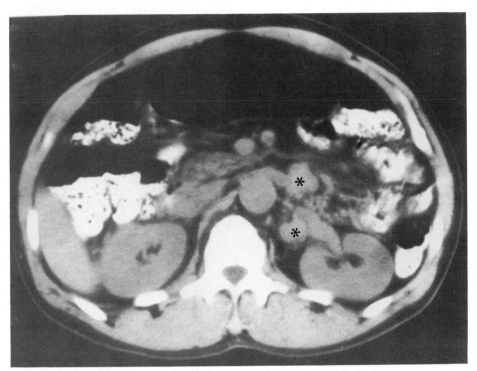

Figure 4–145 Priscilla Lazardi, CT scan at midrenal level.

Karen Weston: *(Continued from page 339)* Figure 4–146 is the lateral view of a subtraction arteriogram following contrast-medium injection into the left external carotid artery, which supplies the meningeal arteries. Note that the tumor mass (arrows) is very hypervascular, well circumscribed, and supplied by meningeal branches of the external carotid artery.

Meningiomas are nearly always hypervascular at angiography and are supplied by meningeal branches of the external carotid arteries. Arteriography may be performed for two reasons: (1) to confirm the nature of the lesion by identification of the blood supply and (2) to embolize these lesions preoperatively to decrease the likelihood of bleeding at surgery.

End of Case

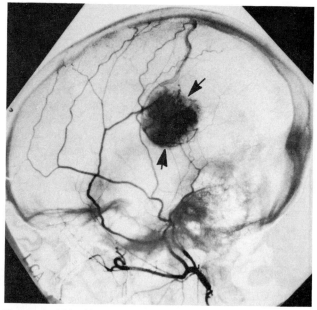

Figure 4–146 Karen Weston, subtraction arteriogram, lateral view.

SMOKER (Continued from Part D, page 340)

Paul Robertson: *(Continued from page 340)* Because of the innumerable collateral vessels that develop when the superior vena cava is occluded, a percutaneous biopsy would be contraindicated because of possibly excessive and uncontrollable bleeding. Therefore, in a more controlled setting, mediastinoscopy with biopsy would be a preferable diagnostic procedure with which to make a diagnosis. In this case, the liver lesion was biopsied. It showed metastatic small cell carcinoma from a primary lung site.

The patient received radiation therapy and improved temporarily, with regression of the initial presenting symptoms of redness and swelling of the face and upper extremities.

End of Case

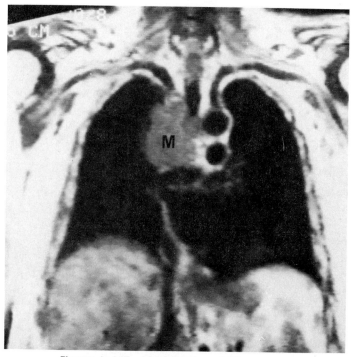

Figure 4–147 Mr. Robertson, MRI scan.

PATIENT WITH HEMATURIA (Continued from Part D, page 343)

Bruce Gunzel: *(Continued from page 343)* An inferior vena cavagram would be the best method of examining this patient. The lateral view shows invasion of the inferior vena cava itself by tumor at the entrance of the renal vein (arrows, Fig. 4–148). MRI can also be used for staging of renal cell carcinoma and defining the inferior vena cava and renal veins.

With the knowledge that the inferior vena cava was involved, the surgeon then removed the large, bulky, tumor-laden right kidney, which was almost completely replaced by tumor. Knowing ahead of time about the inferior vena caval extension, the surgeon utilized a thoracoabdominal approach, cross clamping the inferior vena cava and removing the tumor clot first. Mr. Gunzel had an uneventful recovery, and three months later, in September, returned to teach biology to his favorite junior students.

End of Case

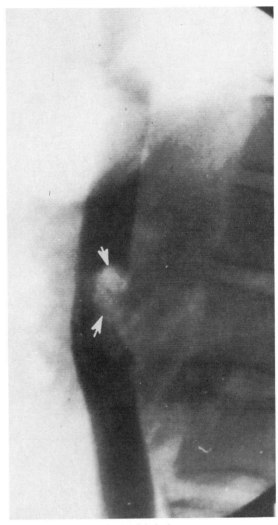

Figure 4–148 Bruce Gunzel, inferior vena cavagram, lateral view.

SWIM COACH WITH KNEE PAIN (Continued from Part D, page 345)

Barbara Crane: *(Continued from page 345)* Either primary or secondary neoplastic bony lesions may occur. Metastatic bone lesions from primary sites, most commonly lung, colon, stomach, breast, and kidney, are relatively common but unlikely in a 20-year-old patient. Usually, these lesions affect the more proximal skeleton, proximal to the knees and elbows. Multiple myeloma and round cell tumors such as lymphoma also tend to cause lytic lesions. Primary bone tumors arise from the basic cells that make up the skeletal structures, that is, osteocytes, chondrocytes, and fibrocytes. They may be either benign or malignant. At the end of a bone, a giant cell tumor, which is a primary bone tumor, has the appearance that you see on Ms. Crane's films. This in fact was proved by biopsy. The giant cell tumor was resected and a bone graft placed in the proximal tibia. A giant cell tumor, although histologically benign, frequently recurs. Ms. Crane went back to instructing her students at the pool.

End of Case

Part F

PATIENT WITH ACUTE BACK PAIN (Continued from Part E, page 346)

Matilda Mason: *(Continued from page 346)* A thoracic aortogram shows a localized aneurysm of the descending portion of the aorta (arrows, Fig. 4–149). The intraluminal contrast medium opacifies the lumen and the aneurysm itself but not the mediastinal hematoma, which was better seen on the CT scan. Mrs. Mason underwent resection of the descending portion of the aorta and was found to have a mycotic aneurysm that was cultured as *Enterobacter*. She recovered uneventfully.

End of Case

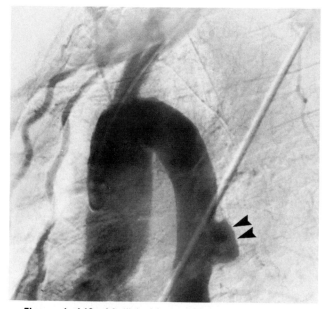

Figure 4–149 Matilda Mason, thoracic arteriogram.

PATIENT WITH GI BLEEDING (Continued from Part E, page 349)

Abner Lane: *(Continued from page 349)* Two days after stopping vasopressin, he should have a barium enema to rule out a colon cancer, polyp, or other lesion that *might* have caused the bleeding masquerading as a bleeding diverticulum. Such a lesion would require further therapy. Mr. Lane's barium enema is done and shows only diverticulosis of the colon, and he is discharged home.

End of Case

Index

Note: Page numbers in *italics* refer to illustrations.

Mammography, breast cancer on, 300, *300*
"Marble bones," 222, 224
Margins, in radiography, 2
Mastectomy, spread of cancer following, *30*, 32, 323, *323*
Mediastinal biopsy, 340
  conditions contraindicating, 352
Mediastinal lymphadenopathy, *260*, 278, *278*, 302, *302*
Mediastinal mass, *19*, 21, *35*, 37, *74–77*, *76*, *260*, 278, *278*, 294, 319
  biopsy in diagnosis of, 340
    conditions contraindicating, 352
  MRI appearance of, 340, *340*, 352
Mediastinal shift, 25, *46*, *47*, 49
  inhaled foreign body and, 308, *309*
Melanoma, 271
  metastasis of, to brain, 293, 317, *317*
    to lungs, 327
Meningioma, 293, 318, 339, *339*, 352, *352*
  symptoms of, 271
Metallic artifacts, on abdominal radiography, *283*, 306
Metaphysis, *214*, 217, 218, *218*
Metastasis. See *Cancer, spread of.*
Middle lobe pneumonia, *26*, 28, *28*, *46*, 49
Miller-Abbott tube, in evaluation of small bowel obstruction, 128, *128*
Modeling, of bone, *219*
  abnormal, *220*, 221, *222*, 224
Morquio's disease, 205, *205*
"Mouse" ("joint mouse"), 200, *200*
MRI (magnetic resonance imaging), abdominal aortic aneurysm on, 288, *289*
  cerebral abscess on, 316, *316*
  cerebral metastatic tumors on, 317, *317*
  fetus on, 102, *103*
  iliac artery aneurysm on, 288, *289*
  mediastinal mass on, 340, *340*, 352
  meningioma on, 339, *339*
Multiple epiphyseal dysplasia, *223*, 225
Multiple gestation, *103*
Multiple myeloma, 338–339
  bone lesions associated with, *194*, 196, *292*, 315, *338*, 339
  patient history in, 270
Mycotic aortic aneurysm, 327, *327*, 346
Myeloma, multiple. See *Multiple myeloma.*
Myocardial infarction, abdominal symptoms associated with, 152
  x-ray findings in, *31*, 32, *45*, 48, *67*, 69, *69*

Neoplasms (tumors). See site-specific entries (e.g., *Bone, tumors of*); *Cancer*; and particular tumor types.
Nephropathy. See *Renal* entries.
Neurological symptoms, chest x-rays in patients presenting with, 62, *63*, 64, *65*, *65*
  computed tomography in patients presenting with, 293
Nodule(s), pulmonary, *18*, *19*, *20*, 21
  cancer appearing as, *18*, *19*, *20*, 21, *263*, 280, 305, *305*, 327
  septic infarcts appearing as, *304*, 326, *326*
Non-Hodgkin's lymphoma, and mediastinal adenopathy, 302, *302*
Nonossifying fibroma, of tibia, *190*, 192
Nutrient canal, of bone, *214*

Obstructive pulmonary disease, chronic, *294*, 319
Ollier's disease (dyschondroplasia, enchondromatosis), *194*, 196, *223*, 225
Ossification. See *Bone growth.*
  centers, 212
  primary, 212, *212*
  secondary, 212, 218
Osteoarthritis (degenerative joint disease), *198*, 200, *200*, *240*, 242, 246–247, *251*, 255
Osteoarthropathy, hypertrophic, *183*, 185
Osteoblastic activity, on radionuclide bone scan, 197
Osteogenesis imperfecta, 205, *205*, *233*, 235
Osteogenic sarcoma, of femur, *191*, 193, *193*, *240*, 242
  of humerus, *183*, 185
Osteoid osteoma, of femur, *182*, 184
Osteomyelitis, *182*, 184, *232*, 234
  tuberculous, *237*, 239
  vs. bone tumor, *241*, 243
Osteopetrosis, 222, 224, *249*, 254
Osteoporosis, 186, *186*, *187*, 188, *189*, *204*, 205
  and fracture, 247
  in hyperparathyroidism, *187*, 189, *189*, 337, *337*
  in osteogenesis imperfecta, 205, *205*, *233*, 235
  in rheumatoid arthritis, 254
  in scurvy, *227*, 229
Ovarian cyst, *101*, 102

Paget's disease, of bone, *178*, 180, *232*, 234
Pain, abdominal, associated with epilepsy, 123
  bone, due to multiple myeloma, 338
  knee, from fracture due to tibial giant cell tumor, 276, 322. See also *Giant cell tumor, of tibia.*
Pancoast tumor, 80, 81
Pancreas, calcifications in, *117*, 118, *118*, 142, *142*, 144, *144*
  cancer of, 321, *321*, 344
    jaundice associated with, 275
  enlarged, 118, *118*
  inflammation of, 283, *283*
    gallstones and, 306
  trauma to, 335, *335*
Pancreatic duct, dilation of, 297, *298*
Pancreatitis, 283, *283*
  gallstones and, 306
Paralytic ileus, vs. mechanical obstruction, *128*, 128–129, *129*
Pathological conditions, categories of, 277
Pelvis, abscess in, *115*, 115
  fracture of, *197*, 198
  in Ollier's disease, *223*, 225
Peptic ulcer, duodenal, 99, *99*. See also *Duodenal ulcer.*
Perforated viscus, signs of, on abdominal radiography, *116*, 118, *135*, 136, *137*, *151*, 152, *153*
  on chest radiography, *14*, 16, *17*, *39*, 41, *83*
Pericardial calcification, *67*, 69, *69*, 83
Pericardial cyst, 75, *76*, 77
Pericardial effusion, *260*, 278, 303, *303*
Pericarditis, *67*, 69, *69*, 303
Periosteum, bone arising from, *182*, *183*, 184, 185, 193, *193*
Peritoneal fluid (ascites), 119, *119*, *130*, 132

Visceral perforation, signs of, on abdominal
radiography, *116*, 118, *135*, 136, *137*,
151, 152, *153*
on chest radiography, *14*, 16, *17*, *39*, 41,
83
Vitamin C deficiency, effects of, *227*, 229
Vitamin D deficiency, and rickets, *178*, 180,
227, 229
Vitamin D treatment, and improvement of
rickets, *229*
Volvulus, cecal, *130*, 132, *134*, 136, *282*, 306,
329, 347, *347*
patient history in, 265

Volvulus *(Continued)*
sigmoid, *105*, 107, *107*

Wheeze, 295
in patient with lung cancer, 273, 295
Wrist, *181*, *184*
atrophy of disuse of, *179*, 181
osteomyelitis involving, *182*, 184
tumor at, *241*, 243

X-ray studies. See *Radiography*.